Francesco Algarotti

The philosophy of Sir Isaac Newton

Francesco Algarotti

The philosophy of Sir Isaac Newton

ISBN/EAN: 9783741104268

Manufactured in Europe, USA, Canada, Australia, Japa

Cover: Foto ©ninafisch / pixelio.de

Manufactured and distributed by brebook publishing software (www.brebook.com)

Francesco Algarotti

The philosophy of Sir Isaac Newton

THE
CONTENTS.

DIALOGUE I.

INTRODUCTION; *a general idea of physics, and an explication of the most remarkable hypotheses concerning* Light and Colours,   page 18

DIALOGUE II.

That qualities, such as Light, Colours, *and the like, are not really in bodies. Metaphysical doubts concerning our sensations of them. Explication of the general principles of Optics,*   57

DIALOGUE III.

Several particulars relating to Vision, discoveries in Optics, and a confutation of the Cartesian *system,*   97

DIALOGUE IV.

Encomium on experimental philosophy, and an exposition of the Newtonian system of Optics,   142

DIALOGUE V.

Exposition of the Newtonian *philosophy continued.* 187

DIALOGUE VI.

Exposition of the Newtonian *universal principle of attraction, and application of this principle to Optics,*   223

TO
Monf. de FONTENELLE.

IF you addreſſed your ingenious and entertaining Dialogues to the illuſtrious Dead, who had firſt given you the idea of that work, and therefor thought yourſelf obliged to ſeek your Hero even in the obſcurity of the tomb; how much greater reaſon have I to dedicate theſe diſcourſes to one of the moſt illuſtrious among the Living, whom I am indebted to for the example which ſet me upon compoſing them, and who has given me ſo perfect a model of polite wit and agreeable writing?

Your Plurality of Worlds firſt ſoftened the ſavage nature of philoſophy, and called it from the ſolitary cloſets and libraries of the learned, to introduce it into the circles and toilets of ladies. You first interpreted to the moſt amiable part of the univerſe thoſe hieroglyphics, which were at firſt only for initiates; and found a happy method to imbelliſh and interſperſe with moſt beautiful flowers a field, which once ſeemed incapable of producing any thing but the moſt rugged thorns and perplexing difficulties. You may be ſaid to have committed the care of revolving the heavens to Venus, and the Graces, inſtead of thoſe intelligences to whom ignorance had anciently aſſigned that office.

The ſucceſs was anſwerable to the beauty and novelty of the undertaking. That half of our world, which always commands the votes of the other, has given its approbation to your book, and in the moſt agreeable manner conſecrated it to poſterity.

May I venture to flatter myſelf, that my Light and Colours will have the ſame fate as your Worlds? If a deſire of pleaſing thoſe who afford us ſo much pleasure, were sufficient to make its fortune, I should have nothing to envy you. But I am too sensible of the very many defects that attend my performance, defects that I cannot help lamenting; for not to say any thing of your talents, and that happy art of rendering every thing you undertake entertaining and agreeable, the plurality of Worlds, which you have chosen for your subject, seems of all others to present the most pleasing and elegant images, and is therefor the most agreeable to your dialogists, that the vast field of philosophy could ever supply you with. It presents to the mind nothing less than the stars and planets, the noblest and most shining objects of the universe. There are but few of the subtile enquiries of science, into which you are obliged to enter. The arguments, upon which your opinion is founded, do not carry such a certainty in them, as to make the conversation grow languid.

I have endeavoured to set truth, accompanied with all that is neceſſary to demonſtrate it, in a pleaſing light, and to render it agreeable to that ſex, which had rather perceive than underſtand. Light and Colours are the ſubject of my dialogues; a ſubject, which, however lively and agreeable it may ſeem, is not in itſelf either ſo pleaſing or ſo extenſive as your worlds. I am obliged to deſcend to many difficult and minute particulars of knowlege; and my arguments are unhappily inconteſtible experiments, which muſt be explained with the greateſt accuracy imaginable. It was indeed juſt, that the ladies, who by your work had been made acquainted with the great change introduced by Des Cartes into the thinking world, ſhould not be ignorant of the new, and, it is probable, the laſt change, of which the illuſtrious Sir Iſaac Newton was the author. But it was extremely difficult to recivilize this ſavage philoſophy, which in the paths of calculation and the moſt abſtruſe Geometry was returning more than ever to its ancient auſterity. You have embelliſhed the Carteſian philoſophy; and I have endeavoured to ſoften the Newtonian, and render its very ſeverities agreeable.

However, the abſtruſe points, upon which I have been obliged to treat, were only ſuch as are abſolutely neceſſary, and always interſperſed with ſomething that may relieve the mind from that attention which they require. In the moſt delightful walk we are ſometimes glad to find a verdant turf to repoſe ourſelves upon. Lines and mathematical figures are entirely excluded, as they would have given theſe diſcourſes too ſcientific an air, and appeared formidable to thoſe, who to be inſtructed muſt be pleaſed. Mathematical terms are as much as poſſible avoided; and if ever any do occur, they are explained by the aſſiſtance of the moſt familiar objects. The difficulties raised against any particular experiment, the history of optical inventions, metaphysical doubts, and the various opinions of different philosophers, preserve the subject from that continued uniformity, which would make it disagreeable and tedious. I have endeavoured as much as possible to render it lively, and make my readers interest themselves in it as they would in a composition for the theatre. Is there any thing, especially where ladies are concerned, in which a writer should omit any endeavours to move the heart?

The marvellous, of which the heart, always desirous of being affected, is so fond, happily arises in true philosophy of itself, without the help of machines. I have made a sort of change or catastrophe in the philosophy of my Marchioness, who is at first a Cartesian, afterwards a proselyte to Malebranche, and at last obliged to embrace the system of that person, who ought to be placed at the head of his species, if superiority and rank among mankind were determined by strength of genius and the most comprehensive knowlege. This great philosopher's general system of attraction is not omitted, because it has a natural connexion with the particular attraction observed betwixt bodies and light. Thus these dialogues may be considered as a complete treatise of the Newtonian philosophy. The sanctuary of the temple will always be reserved for the priests and favourites of the Deity; but the entrance and its other less retired parts will be open to the profane.

The stile I have endeavoured to follow is what I believed most proper for dialogue, clear, concise, interrupted, or intersperfed with images or turns of wit. I have taken the utmost care to avoid those perplexed and long periods closed by the verb, which only serve to run the reader out of breath, and are beside repugnant to good sense, and much less agreeable to the genius of our language than is generally believed, and certainly cannot be agreeable to the genius of those, who write with an intention of being understood. I have left them entirely to those, who forsake the *Saggiatore for the †Fiammetta, together with those antique and obsolete words which constitute so great a part both of their knowlege and delight. The Count di Castiglione, in his Courtier, two centuries ago, ventured to write in such a manner, as to be understood by his contemporaries, and throwing aside the affectation of Gothic terms, adapted his manner of writing to the forms of speech in use among the polite and well-bred persons of his time. Custom the sovereign judge in all languages, except perhaps our own, was his guide; and thus he enriches us with the finest piece, as far

---

* An Epistle from *Galileo* to *Virginius Cesarinus*, in which the author gives a very elegant exposition of his system of Physics and Astronomy.
† A Romance, by *Boccace*.

as regards the style, which the Italian language has to boast of. For what reason should I think myself obliged to make use of the antiquated discourses of some clamorous haranguer of four hundred years standing, as a model for a work of philosophy and politeness; and rather than talk to ladies in the language of the present age, address my discourse to the devotees of the thirteenth century?

This minute dissertation I thought in some measure due to yourself, to let you see how little I have neglected in a manner of writing, which may be regarded as your own. Nor was it less due to my countrymen, since this work, whatever it be, is written in their original language. Young mathematicians, in giving the solution of a problem, generally describe the steps by which they investigated it: it is only those of an established reputation who are permitted to give the simple solution, and leave to others the care of finding by what means they attained it.

I would not however appear to set a greater value upon this work than perhaps the world will think it deserves, or suppose myself to have given a perfect solution of this problem. I am too well acquainted both with myself, and the difficulty of the enterprize, to entertain so high an opinion of the performance. I have perhaps only seen the method, which ought to be followed, and yet have not followed it myself. Raphael and Guercino had nearly an equal knowlege of the preparations necessary for the right designing of a figure, and yet were extremely unequal in the execution of it.

Whatever may be the success of my undertaking, the ladies, for whom this work is principally intended, ought at least to think themselves obliged to me, if I have procured to them a new kind of amusement, which others may perhaps carry to a greater degree of perfection; and if I have brought into

Italy a new mode of cultivating the mind, rather than the preſent momentary faſhon of adjuſting their head-dreſs and placing their curls. Travellers ſhould be the importers of wit, and of thoſe reciprocal advantages, which different nations even in this reſpect have over each other. Happy the ſociety formed upon the Italian fancy, the French politeneſs, and Britiſh good ſenſe!

We ought to think ourſelves obliged to your nation, and yourſelf in particular, for giving us an example to render common and eaſy what was once myſterious and difficult, and to write in our own language what by a ſuperſtitious veneration was appropriated to the Latin, and at the ſame time perplexed with Greek, that moſt formidable weapon of pedantry. We may in this reſpect caſt the ſame reproach on the Italians as Mr. Pope does in another caſe on the Engliſh in his fine prologue to Cato.

Our ſcene precariouſly ſubſiſts too long
On French *tranſlation and* Italian *ſong.*

Dare to have sense yourselves, assert the stage,
Be justly warm'd with your own native rage.

If we except some translations from the French, there is nothing among us but songs and collections of verses, which every day overspread us like a deluge, and are the torments of our age. In the modern books, written in the Italian language, the ladies can find nothing but sonnets full of a metaphysical love, which I suppose must affect them as little as the antiquated expressions of superannuated Cicisbei. Let the age of realities once more arise among us, and knowlege instead of giving a rude and savage turn to the mind, and exciting endless disputes and wrangling upon some obsolete phrase, serve to polish and adorn society. I have at least opened the way to something, which is neither grammar nor sonnet; and I shall flatter myself to have done much more, if what the ladies inspired me with, has the good fortune to meet with your approbation.

ON LIGHT and COLOURS.

DIALOGUE I.

A general idea of Physics, and an explanation of the most remarkable hypotheses concerning Light *and* Colours.

THE very same reason that led me every day to a concert of music, a gay and elegant entertainment, a ball or the theatre, induced me to write an account of the manner in which I passed my time last summer in the country with the marchioness of E——, and has thus, from an idle and useless member of society, rendered me an author. And the natural desire that every author has to appear in print (whatever these gentlemen may tell us in their long prefaces) engages me at present to publish this account. It is entirely philosophical, and composed of certain discourses which I had with that polite lady on the subject of Light and Colours. Some will, I make no doubt, condemn me for having passed my time so ill with a lady; and indeed I have condemned myself for it. But if they knew what an engaging manner the marchioness has of obliging every one to what she desires, I am persuaded they would forgive me, even if I had read her Guicciardini's * history of the wars of Pisa, if she could have desired it. But however inexcusable my error might be, I constantly endeavoured to amend it, whenever I could

---

* An Italian historian very prolix and tedious. It was a saying of Dr. Donne's, that if Moses had wrote like Guicciardini, the whole world would not have been big enough to contain the history of its own creation.

disengage myself a little from Light and Colours, and indeed both the beauty of the marchioness, and the nature of the place, which seemed formed to support what she had every where given birth to, inspired a discourse quite different from that of philosophy. The little peninsula of Sirmione, the country of the polite Catullus, and those mountains which have so often repeated the fine verses of Fracastorius *, two remarkable points, if I may use the expression, in the poetical geography, formed a distant prospect to a fine seat, placed on an easy ascent, that was watered below with the clear streams of the Benaco †, which by its great extent, and the roring of its waves, seems to rival the ocean. The orange trees that diffused their odours along the banks, and perfumed the air all around with a delightful fragrance, the coolness of the woods, the murmur of fountains, the vessels that spread their sails along the chrystal lake, each of these agreeable objects would have alternately ravished my senses, if the goddess of this delightful place had not wholly engaged my attention.

To the charms of wit, and the most polite imagination she joined an uncommon strength of judgment, and to the most refined sentiments a learned curiosity. Superior to the rest of her sex, without being solicitous to appear so,

---

* Jerom Fracastorius was born of a noble family at Verona in Italy, about the year 1483. He studied physic, until a few years before his death, when he devoted himself entirely to the study of polite learning, mathematics, astronomy, and cosmography. He died of an apoplexy in 1553, and was interred in the church of St Euphemia at Verona, where in 1559, he had a statue erected to him by order of that city. His poetical works are much admired, the principal of which are his *Syphilis*; *Joseph* an epic poem in two books, but left unfinished at his death; and his *Alcon, seu de cura canum venaticorum*. See his life prefixed to his works; *Joann. Imperialis musæum historicum.* pag 16. *Les eloges des hommes savans, tirez de l' histoire de M. de Thou*. Tom. i. pag. 189.

† A lake in in the territories of Venice, now called *Lago di Garda*.

she could talk of ornament and dress whenever there was occasion for it, and ask proper questions upon more important subjects. A natural negligence, an easy unaffectedness, embellished all she said. She had beauty enough to gain her consort many friends, and judicious enough not to shew any one a particular regard; and these accomplishments being seldom found united except in books and the imagination of authors, is the reason, I believe, that learning in ladies does not meet with so universal an applause from the world as their beauty.

When impertinent visitors gave us some respite from play, that relief and plague of society, we passed some part of the day in reading ancient and modern authors, contrary to the opinion of that monarch * who preferred old books like old friends. Our principal reading was poetry, as this seemed of all others most agreeable to the country from whence the genealogists of polite literature tell us it derived its original. But, however, that we might preserve a certain spirit of liberty, upon which all our conversation was grounded, we did not entirely exclude that sort of poetry which is formed expresly for the town, as satire, comedy, and epic. This spirit had a more particular influence upon our criticism, which regarded an Italian, a French, an ancient and a modern author, with an equal impartiality. The sober dignity and purity of the Eneid, the variety and perspicuity of Orlando Furioso, the noble finishing of the Gierusalemme Liberata, the justness, the philosophical spirit, and the

* Alphonsus the 10th king of *Arragon*, sirnamed the Wise, who used to say, he desired little more than four *old* things, *viz. old* wood to burn, *old* wine to drink, *old* books to read, and *old* friends to live with. He began his reign in 1252, and died in 1284.

peculiar beauties of the Henriade, the invention of the Mandragora *, the characters of the Misanthrope, the sweetness of verse in † Sannazarius, and the happy negligence of Chappelle; all these we compared in such a manner, that we neither esteemed a verse the more harmonious for its antiquity, nor a thought less sublime or elegant from any difference of country. We interspersed our discourse with episodes and digressions, which the marchioness did not think herself less obliged to me for, than if I had given her an encomium upon her beauty.

In one of these digressions, I spoke of the force and advantages of English poetry, which gave her a strong inclination to be acquainted with it, imagining that a nation, to whom Minerva had lavished her favours in so profuse a manner, could not be destitute of those of Apollo.

As I desired nothing more than to give pleasure to a person who continually afforded so much to me, I was extremely sorry that I could trace her only a very low and imperfect idea of Dryden's harmonious copiousness, Waller's softness, Prior's various and easy stile, the lively wit and fire of Rochester and Dorset, the correct majesty of Addison, the strong and manly strokes of Shakespeare,

---

* Mandragora or Mandragola, an Italian comedy written by the famous Nicolas Machiavel.

† Actius Sincerus Sannazarius was born at Naples of a noble family in 1488. He was secretary to Ferdinand king of Naples, who honoured him with a great share of his confidence and esteem. He was eminent for his Italian and Latin verses. He spent twenty years in correcting and polishing his poem *De Partu Virginis* ; but his piscatory Eclogues in *Latin*, which he wrote when he was young, were preferred to all his other poetical writings. He was rewarded by the Venetians with a present of 600 crowns for his celebrated epigram,

Viderat Hadriacis Venetam, etc.

He died in 1530 of grief, because the prince of Orange, who was general of the imperial army, had demolished a tower belonging to his country-house. He lies interred near Virgil's tomb. See *Paulus Jovius in Elogiis*, etc.

and the astonishing sublimity of Milton. To speak of the merit of a poet, is the same thing as endeavouring to describe the beauty of a face, which can be judged of only by the sight; and to quote, even in its original language, only one particular passage separate from the rest, would be the same as shewing an eye, a lip, or a dimple of a face, of which we desire to see not single features, but the whole, whose beauty and symmetry are the result of innumerable charms. However it gave me a little consolation when I remembered, that, among some papers which I happened to bring with me into the country, I had Mr. Pope's Ode on St. Cecilia's day. None can be unacquainted with the name of this great author, without at the same time ignorant that there is any such thing as poetry in the *English* language. The next morning I carried this fine Ode with me into the grove dedicated to our poetical conversation, and now become the Parnassus of all nations. After having begged pardon of the *English* muses, I translated it as well as I could, and began to read. The marchioness listened to me with an attention that fine ladies seldom give themselves the trouble of. When I came to this passage——

While in more lengthen'd notes and slow *
The deep majestic solemn organs blow;

she interrupted me, and could not enough admire the propriety of these *epithets*, which, added she, describe that instrument in such a manner that I really hear it play. I cannot tell whether you hear it too, but I think I may reasonably conclude it from a certain pleasure you shewed, perhaps, insensibly, in reading this passage to me. You

---
* Mentre con tarde ed allungate note
Il profundo, solenne, e maestoso
Organo soffia ——

are so well acquainted, Madam, with the most secret motions of my heart, that it is impossible for you to be deceived; and you commend a thing that certainly renders the image, which is the support of poetry, extremely lively and expressive. These sorts of *epithets* are the strokes that give life to the picture. A *white* hand, a *serene* brow, and *bright* eyes, are at best but the rough draught of it.

Now we are speaking of epithets, is not *the seven-fold Light*, which I read of some time ago, replied the marchioness, in an Ode made in honour of the philosophical lady * of Bologna, some Chinese hieroglyphic? at least it is so to me and many others whom I have desired to explain it. You mean, answered I,

——*The* sevenfold *Light*
Whence ev'ry pleasing charm of colour springs,
And forms the gay variety of things †.

If you knew the force of this epithet, you would see a Newtonian picture instead of a Chinese hieroglyphic, though perhaps a little too philosophical for poetry. What! answered she, interrupting me with an air of surprize, you understand this passage as well, as if it was the production of an English author. I am of opinion, Madam, answered I, that the verses of an Italian who has the honour to be a great admirer of you, are infinitely preferable to those of an unfortunate Briton, who has the unhappiness of being at so great a distance from you. I understand you, continued she, and I need not desire a better

---

* Laura Maria Katherina Barsi, a learned lady in Italy, who in 1732, at 19 years old, held a philosophical disputation at Bologna, upon which she was admitted to the degree of doctor in that university.

† O dell' aurata
Luce settemplice
I varioardenti, e misti almi colori.

encomiaſt than you, if it be true, that no one underſtands the ſenſe of an author ſo well as himſelf. Come then, ſince you are the author of this piece, deliver me from the perplexity I am under about this *ſevenfold* Light, and the reſt of your Newtonian picture, which gives me great reaſon to believe, that in praiſing one lady, you have uſed your utmoſt endeavours that no other ſhould underſtand your meaning. It is certainly that profound reſpect that I have for you, Madam, anſwered I, which has made you find me out. Afterwards, reflecting that it was impoſſible to give her in few words an explication of Sir Iſaac Newton's optics to which theſe verſes allude, a thing which ſhe had not the leaſt idea of, had not we better follow the example of the theatre, Madam, ſaid I, where the play is generally at an end when the perſons come to a knowlege of one another? And beſides, we ſhould finiſh Mr. Pope's Ode, which will certainly give you a far greater pleaſure, than any comment upon mine. No, no, ſaid ſhe, we will finiſh that another time, and for the preſent we ſhall act contrary to the theatre, but without forgetting the cataſtrophe, or finding myſelf in as much ignorance as ever.

Being willing to give her ſome idea of the ſyſtem to which theſe verſes refer, and thinking that the Marchioneſs would for once be like other ladies, who are often deſirous of ſeeming to underſtand what they are not ſuppoſed to have the leaſt notion of, I told her as briefly as I could, that according to Sir Iſaac Newton's opinion, or rather as the thing really is, every ray of light is compoſed of in infinite number of other rays, ſome of which are red, ſome orange and yellow colour, others green, ſome blue, ſome indigo, and others violet; and that from the compoſition of theſe ſeven colours in a direct ray from the ſun ariſes the white or rather golden colour of light: that if this direct ray from the sun is refracted by a certain glass called a prism, these rays of which it is composed, differing in colour, differ also in degrees of refrangibility.——I see, said the marchioness, interrupting me in a manner very different from what I expected, that your comment has more need of an explanation than perhaps the text itself. But this is my fault in not being able to understand your *refraction, different degrees of refrangibility*, and the like, which quite confound the idea I had begun to form. But pray explain yourself in such a manner that I may not have any farther reason to accuse you with obscurity, nor my own dulness with being the cause of it.

You will not be satisfied, answered I, unless I make you a comment at least as long as that of the Malmantile, which, I observed to you the other day, seemed to be dictated by the agreeable Mathanasius * who was formerly the Moliere of the commentators: at least, said she, Newton will enter more properly here than Micheli does there, whose discoveries are of no sort of service to illustrate this poem; and since all you said was spoke with an air of seriousness, and such confidence that you did not scruple saying, *according to* Sir Isaac Newton's *opinion, or rather as the thing really is*, you have made me extremely desirous of becoming a Newtonian. This, answered I, is a very ready method of propagating Sir Isaac Newton's philosophy and bringing it into fashion. Pemberton, Gravesand, and Dunch, the zealous propagators of this

---

* Monsieur de St. Hyacinthe, under the fictitious name of Dr. Mathanasius, published a piece intitled, *Chef d'Oeuvre d'un Inconnu avec des remarques*, in order to ridicule the impertinence of some critics and commentators. The *Malmantile* is an Italian piece wrote after the manner of this author.

ſyſtem, would be very glad to give the care of it to you. But what will Mr. Pope ſay, ſhewing her the book which I had ſtill in my hand, if you leave him in the beginning of this fine Ode, for a ſudden fancy that you have taken to light and colours? Mr. Pope, anſwered ſhe, cannot be offended at my leaving him for a philoſopher, and ſuch a philoſopher as Sir Iſaac Newton, one of his own countrymen too. Do not you know, ſaid I ſmiling, that the poets look upon themſelves as ſacred, and when they have once got this enthuſiaſm into their heads, they regard neither country nor relations, but think themſelves greater than any philoſopher, even if he had diſcovered wherein conſiſts the union of the ſoul and body? It is well for us, ſaid ſhe, that the poets have more modeſty than to declare this in their writings.

It ſignified nothing for me to plead incapacity and many other excuſes, which are made uſe of on the like occaſions, and which occurred to me upon this. The marchioneſs inſiſted upon ſeeing my Newtonian picture as ſhe called it. I begged ſhe would at leaſt have patience till evening, telling her that the night had always been the time conſecrated to philoſophical affairs; and that the moſt polite philoſopher in France had made uſe of it in a circumſtance reſembling mine, and made no ſcruple of entertaining a fine lady with philoſophical diſcourſes in a wood at midnight. But we, Sir, replied the marchioneſs, ought to make uſe of the day, which is certainly more proper than the night for a diſcourſe on light and colours. She ſpoke this with an air of authority that inforced her commands in the moſt amiable manner, and made it a pleaſure to obey.

Thus I was abſolutely obliged to begin, but the diffi-

culty was how to do it; for she had not the least notion
of physics, which it was necessary to give her a general
idea of, before I proceeded to a discourse upon light and
colours on the Newtonian system. At last, after having
again in vain reminded her of Mr. Pope, and other subjects
that required less application and afforded greater pleasure, when the heat of the sun, which was now almost at
his meridian, obliged us to retire into the house, I began
after the following manner.

It is natural to suppose that after society was so well established among mankind, that some of them had nothing
to do, which I look upon as the epocha of its perfection.
These persons either from that curiosity, which we naturally have about those things that concern us least, or
perhaps for fear of being charged with idleness by the rest,
applied themselves to consider that variety of things of
which this universe is composed, their differences and effects. It is probable too, that one of the first speculations
that these idle people, who afterwards assumed the name
of *philosophers*, employed themselves about, was concerning the nature of light, which is certainly the most beautiful and conspicuous object of our sight, and indeed the
means by which we see every thing else. This consequently led them to the colours which this light depictures
upon objects, and which diffuse such a variety and beauty
on our world. Thus, I believe, that *Optics*, which is
that part of natural philosophy that regards light and
colours, and in general all natural philosophy, had their
origin among men at the same time with their idleness:
indeed it was of a latter date than some parts of morality
and geometry, which were absolutely necessary in the ear-
liest ages of the world, but contemporary to poetry, if

you will, and antecedent to metaphyſics, which required a ſtill greater vacation from buſineſs.

I am pleaſed, replied the marchioneſs, that poetry and natural philoſophy have one common date; ſince for that reaſon you will not perhaps think this tranſition ſo ſtrange, that we have made from one to the other upon my account. The tranſition, anſwered I, that our philoſophers made from a ſlight knowlege of things to an ambition of unfolding nature and penetrating its effects, was much ſtronger. This, in the language of philoſophy, is called making *ſyſtems*. This is juſt as if any one, after having had a curſory diſcourſe with a ſubtile miniſter of ſtate about good or bad weather, ſhould attempt to write his character, and pretend that he had penetrated his moſt profound ſecrets They ſhould have begun with a very attentive examination of things, drawn from frequent obſervations and diligent experiments before they ventured upon the leaſt ſyſtem They were to act, if poſſible, like thoſe two antient philoſophers; one* of whom, in order to write on the nature of bees, retired into a wood, that he might have the better opportunity of conſidering them; and the other † ſpent ſixty years in making obſervations upon theſe inſects. But the misfortune is, that experiments and obſervation require patience and time, and very often we are indebted to mere chance for the muſt uſeful and entertaining among them. On the other hand, men are always in haſte to arrive at knowlege, or at leaſt to have the appearance of it.

After this, the revolutions of ſtates, the rude and uncultivated manners of the people, the temper of nations, and

* Philiſcus. Vid. Plin. N. H. L. xi. C. 9.
† Ariſtomachus. Id. ibid.

the profession of those, among whom philosophy had formerly flourished, did not a little retard its progress. From the Indians traditions which their priests kept to themselves with as much jealousy as they did their genealogies, and from the Egyptian temples, where it had long lain hid under mysteries and hieroglyphics, philosophy at length took its seat in the portico's and gardens of Greece, where it was very soon embellished, and corrupted with allegory, fables, and all the ornaments of eloquence. Imagination, which is the characteristic of the Grecian genius, prevented philosophy from taking any deep root, and indeed it was attempted to have been totally extirpated by the eloquence of a man, whose discourses were distinguished by a certain grave and elegant pleasantry, which made him master of the most powerful arts of persuasion, and who had been judged by the oracle the wisest among mortals. He asserted, that we have nothing to do with what is above us, and strove to reclaim our curiosity and studies from natural to moral objects; from the combinations of the universe, to the little chaos of human extravagancies, and from that rapture with which we are transported by the contemplation of vast and distant objects, to the melancholy consideration of our own emptiness. And this person, who, more destructive than Pandora, engaged mankind in a consideration of that train of evils which had issued from her fatal box, without giving them * any hopes of a cure, was had in the highest veneration, as the father of a new philosophy called *moral*, which is of all others the most treated of and the least understood.

* It is probable that the greater part of those, who are acquainted with the character of Socrates, will think our noble author has passed too severe a censure.

after this, together with luxury, riches, and
s transported from Asia to Rome. It could
 progress among a people who cultivated
er arts but those of pardoning the vanquish-
ssing the proud. In the first ages of chri-
ophy lent its assistance to combat paganism,
was subdued, it raised so many civil wars
 among those who by its assistance had tri-
Jupiter and Olympus, that the ecclesiastical
 danger of perishing when it was hardly
 port. To this fatal war of words suc-
hich the Barbarians raised against learning
n empire, wherein both were equal suffer-
troyed the one, and sunk the other, untill
ound darkness, which afterwards followed,
f antient knowlege were re-kindled among

The doctrine of Aristotle revived, and be-
ough the East, was gladly embraced by the
as the most suitable to their manner of life.
ins and study are necessary to frame a right
 requires no less art and labour, than to
 silks which you ladies are adorned with.
ophy, in which the name of Aristotle sup-
 of reason, did not greatly disturb the mo-
lity. This philosopher, who was banished
by the antient priests, was, but with some

ired from Athens, in order to avoid a process of ir-
he Athenian priests carried on against him. The
 this affair are unknown: some assert, that he was
piety on account of a hymn which he had made in
end Hermius. This hymn is still extant, but there
impiety discoverable in it; but his accusers urged
 haned divine songs by prostituting them to the ho-
l man. Aristotle, not thinking it safe to trust to the
 his little poem might meet with, retired very pri-

C

variety of fortune, received by ours; who, though they
once condemned him as a * pernicious author, yet after
wards carried the zeal for him to such a height, as to believe him not ignorant even of those things which are a-
bove the reach of human reason. Religion at this time
was more than ever united with philosophy, which could
not fail to produce the utmost confusion in the one, and
ignorance in the other, since both their nature and end
are extremely different.

A chaos of vain and useless disputes, a chain of unintelligible definitions, a blind zeal for wrangling, and a still
blinder devotion for Aristotle whom they called, by way of

---

vately to Chalcis, where he pleaded his cause at a distance by writing, which was the safest way he could take; for his accusers were
a set of men who would never have let him been at rest. Others affirm that he was driven from Athens for the goodness of his morals.
Some authors report, that this philosopher drowned himself in the
Euripus, a narrow sea near Eubæa, because he could not find out
the reason of its ebbing and flowing seven times a day. But the more
received opinion is, that his very great application, in the study of
this phænomenon, brought an illness upon him, which occasioned
his death. See Bayle's life of Aristotle in the general dictionary,
vol. II.

* The French, who took Constantinople about the 13th century,
having brought the books of Aristotle into their own country, his
doctrine began to be publickly taught in the university of Paris, and
continued so for some time. But Arnaury a student of that university, having advanced several obnoxious opinions, and endeavoured
to defend them, from the principles of Aristotle, the physics and
metaphysics of that philosopher were burnt by order of a council
held at Paris in 1209, and the reading of them prohibited under pain
of excommunication. This prohibition was confirmed about the
year 1215, by the Pope's legate, who was employed to reform the
university of Paris; but he allowed the logic of Aristotle to be
taught. Gregory VII. renewed this prohibition in 1231, but with
this addition, that he only forbid the reading of Aristotle's works
till they should be corrected. In 1261, Simon the legate of the see
of Rome in his reformation of the university confirmed the regula-
tion of the year 1215, relating to Aristotle's writings without mentioning the correction of them. But in the reformation of the university in 1366, this philosopher's physics, as his other works, were
allowed to be read. Vid. Father Rapin's comparison of Plato and
Aristotle; Du Pin's Nouvelle bibl. etc.

distinction, *the philosopher*, or a second nature, and above all a certain jargon of indeterminate, obscure and hard expressions, either without any meaning, or confused, overspread, like a destroying deluge, the face of the whole earth, and for many ages usurped the pompous name of science. As among the Chinese he is esteemed the most learned, who can read and write more words and figures than the rest, so he was counted to have most learning amongst us, who, in a particular habit, could pronounce in certain places, and with certain gestures, and seemed to understand the greater number of expressions in this vain and pedantic jargon. The distinctions and answers might be as easily foreseen by any one who had a little examined their memoirs, as the turns of music in country scrapers, or the jingling of rhyme in bad poets. Such were the vails under which they hid, from the eyes of the world, that ignorance which very often they could not hide from themselves. The pride of schools was supported by the noise of empty words, and the tyranny of names. It was imagined that they really contended for truth, but these grayheaded children in reality amused themselves only in fighting with bubbles.

This obstinate veneration for the antients, which for a long while passed among the philosophers as hereditary from one generation to another, was the cause that the knowlege of physics made little or no progress till the last age. At length, among some few others, who were to fall as it were martyrs to reason, there appeared in Tuscany a person named * Galileo, who had the courage not

---

* Galileo was born at Florence in 1564. He was put into the inquisition for maintaining the diurnal motion of the earth, and asserting the sun and not the earth to be the center of the world. These propositions were condemned by the Inquisitors as false and heretical. He was not discharged till he had promised to renounce

not only to say, but what is worse, to demonstrate with the clearest evidence, that men, who had perhaps for sixty years been honoured with the title of doctors, or sat in the chair of philosophy, had taken very great pains all their life long to know nothing. All this boldness cost him dear; for to venture to make use of his reason was the same thing as reproaching them with the general abuse they had made of theirs; and to endeavour at the promotion of knowlege was as dangerous as an attempt to change the boundaries of antient Rome, which the Augurs took such a religious care in the preservation of. After such a course of ages, he shewed them what ought to have been done at first, and began to make a search into nature by observations and experiments, reducing himself to that ignorance which is useful for arriving to some knowlege at last.

I think it not improper to call this man the czar, Peter the Great, in natural philosophy: each of them had to do with a nation pretty near the same character. No one people ever used such endeavours for knowlege, as the Muscovites did to know nothing. They forbid all strangers to come into their country, and all the natives to go out of it, for fear they should introduce something new.

---

his opinions, and not to defend them either by word or writing, or insinuate them into the mind of any person. Upon his publishing his dialogues upon the two chief systems of the world, the Copernican and Ptolemaic in 1632. he was again cited before the holy office. The same year the congregation convened, and in his presence pronounced sentence against him and his book, committing him to the prison of the holy office during pleasure, and commanding him as a saving penance for three years to come and repeat once a week the seven penitential psalms, but reserving to themselves the power of moderating, changing, and taking away, altogether or in part, the above mentioned punishment and penance. He was discharged from his confinement, in 1634, but the impression of his dialogues of the system of the world was burnt at Rome. Vid. the general dictionary.

Thus was it with these philosophers, who, jealous of their tenets, renounced every experiment, and more certain demonstration of the moderns, rather than introduce any novelty or reformation into their own systems: but as force has generally more influence upon men than reason, the Czar compassed his designs sooner than Galileo, who was at the same time obstructed by another species of philosophers, who were by so much the more formidable as they too despised the antients, which now began to be the fashion, and asserted things in opposition to them of which every one had a clear and distinct idea. They introduced exactness and order in writing, which were then as uncommon as they are natural and necessary, and by means alone of certain motions and figures, which they knew how to give to bodies at proper times and on proper occasions, promised to unfold what seemed the most unexplicable in nature. You may easily imagine that the magnificent promises of these philosophers, which so agreeably flattered the ambition of the human mind, which Galileo's observations served rather to humble, joined to a certain simplicity that gave such an air of wonder to their systems, as it does to a well concerted romance, must naturally seduce many people, and form a sect. And it indeed had this effect; so that these moderns too began to have expositors, and followers as obstinate and zealous as those of the antients had been before; and these made themselves the more ridiculous by laughing at the same fault in others. But it was a melancholy thing to see an experiment sometimes offer itself, which had never before been known or thought on; and the finest and most artificial systems, which had perhaps cost their inventors whole months of labour and study, shamefully fall to the ground.

32   DIALOGUE I.

In order then to avoid thefe forrowful reflections, faid the marchionefs, it is neceffary for thofe, who would form a fyftem in any thing, to be careful firft to take notice of all that is obfervable in it, that it may not be expofed to the mercy and infults of experiments. This is exactly what the Newtonians fay, anfwered I; and certainly, madam, you muft have fome fecret intelligence with them to be fo well informed of their fentiments. It would be ridiculous for a mechanic to take it in his head, to guefs how the famous clock of Strafbourg is made within fide, if he had not firft acquainted himfelf with the outfide, the manner in which it ftrikes, and thofe many other things it does befides telling the hour. Thus, fay they, if we can ever hope to make fyftems that carry fome appearance of being durable, it will be then only when by the means of experiments and obfervations we fhall know all, that in terms of art is called *phænomenon*, which fignifies the appearance of things, and the laws which refult from thefe phænomena, and by which nature conftantly performs all her operations. How then could Des Cartes, for example, who was the chief author of this enterprifing fect of philofophers, make a rational fyftem concerning *light* and *colours*, when he was entirely ignorant of fo many of their qualities, which Sir Ifaac Newton afterwards difcovered by obfervations? How could he form the ftatue, when he had not the marble? This is the manner in which the reft of the philofophers of our time, and thofe learned focieties, founded and maintained by the liberality of princes, or the genius of nations, proceed: they make obfervations and prepare materials for pofterity to build fyftems upon, more fortunate in their duration, than thofe that preceded the prefent age. This profeffion indeed is not fo pompous as that of those who will build you a world in a twinkling of an eye; but on the other hand it has this advantage, that it is able to make good its promises, which is as great an obligation upon a philosopher, as a mistress.

I, who am a woman, replied the Marchioness, confess that I love those who have the courage to venture upon grand and difficult enterprises. Is not this the reason why we interest ourselves so much in the adventures of heroes? The courage of those philosophical heroes has something sublime and superior in it: if they do not attain to all they promise, must there not be given some indulgence to the imperfections of human nature? On the other hand, if, as you say, there cannot be any good systems, till all the phænomena are fully known, when shall we have them? They will happen as seldom with us, as the secular games anciently among the Romans: and I cannot flatter myself that I shall live long enough to see so much as one in my time. I must be contented then with those systems that we have, be they what they will. I believe, Madam, answered I, that no one could have more specious reasons to allege in favour of trifles. I should serve you right, if I put you on proving these reasons; but as I will act more mercifully with you, than you perhaps would with regard to me, since you have a mind that we should reason away that time, which might be better employed on pleasure, I will not make use of that right which these reasons of yours give me, to propose to you seriously the important questions, whether light be a substance, or an accident, or an act of the pellucid, as far as it is pellucid? Whether colours are the first configurations of matter, or a certain little flame that arises from bodies, whose parts are proportioned to our sight? I might gravely ask you too, that you may see how many things I spare you the trouble of considering at once, whether light, or its spirit, be the soul that Plato places between nature and ideas, to connect the sensible and intellectual world? and whether it was for this reason that Plato represented the element of fire, which is the seat of light, under the figure of a pyramid, which in some measure agrees with that sublime and mystic triangle which is the symbol of the soul? idle enigmas of the learned ignorance of past ages! and who can tell but if you had fallen into other hands than mine, you might have been set a yawning with some gothic passages out of Dante? Or perhaps by this light, you would have been gradually conducted to divinity; at least you could not have got free from an explication of the mystic sense hid under the fable of Prometheus, who stole light from the sun to animate his statue.

I see, said the Marchioness, that philosophers are to be dealt with in a very circumspect manner, who know how to improve every thing to their own advantage. You act just like tyrants, who think they confer a great favour on any one, whom they have not injured. However, I am much obliged to you, for sparing me the trouble of hearing all these fine things, which, I confess, are quite above my understanding.

Let us see, answered I, whether you can understand the doctrines of some among the ancients who were more prudent and humane than the rest. These laboured to explain every thing by a vacuum, and the motion and figure of certain very little particles, which they called atoms, and from thence gave their schools the name of *atomists*, which was perhaps the most antient of all other sects, and lately tried by the splendor of eloquence to rise upon the ruins of the Aristotelian, in opposition to that of Descartes. These philosophers asserted that the light of the sun, for example, was nothing but a perpetual and copious stream, of the very little particles, or atoms, which, flowing from the sun himself, spread themselves every way with an incredible velocity, and fill the immense aerial space; so that light is always followed by new light, and one ray is as it were impelled by a second. You may easily understand this by the similitude of a fountain.—I understand it mighty well, interrupted the Marchioness, without the fountain; but I am greatly afraid that these atomists of yours, by making so many particles continually proceed from the sun, will at last turn some fine day into midnight. Truly, answered I, that would be playing us a villainous trick, which no one would get any thing by, unless perhaps some few beauties, who would then always be seen by candle light: but do not fear it. Revolutions of this importance require more time to be brought about, than the revolution of a monarchy. And besides, these atomists give us so great a security that it would be a shame to dread it. For, in the first place, they tell us, that the rarity and incredible smalness of these little particles that proceed from the sun, which sun they make to be of a dense and close matter as you will see hereafter, in a very long course of years will produce only a very little diminution in his light. And to make you still more secure, this may be confirmed by the example of a little grain of colour, which is sufficient to tinge a very great quantity of water. An example, drawn from odorous bodies, may serve to shew you how very much the parts of matter may be subtilised; as for instance, a grain of musk, which, though it continually emits a prodigious quantity of particles, yielding a perfume so strong and quick, that at a certain distance it is able to stupify serpents of a monstrous size, and quite deprive them of motion, yet in a considerable time its weight is but very little diminished. And amber-grease, in the same manner, for a long while loses hardly any thing of its agreeable scent. From light's passing through the densest bodies, such as diamonds, and gold when it is beaten into thin plates, we must necessarily infer, that the particles of light are extremely subtile. All this is mighty well, replied the Marchioness; but that such a quantity of light should continually proceed from the sun, as is sufficient to fill and illuminate the whole world, puts me into terrible apprehensions, notwithstanding all your fine examples of musk, amber grease, and diamonds.

Have not you some inclination, answered I, to the learned melancholy of the inhabitants of Dean Swift's flying island? who in the most poetical allegories has given us the most philosophical satire upon mankind. This island, which in the language of the country is called Laputa, as it is different from all that have hitherto been discovered by our voyagers, so it is inhabited by a very singular species of men: always abstracted and immersed in the profoundest speculations, they give themselves up to spleen and the mathematics, so that they have always need of a *Flapper*, who, by striking them from time to time with a bladder, may bring them back to the world below; their knowlege fills them with those continual fears and disquietudes which the vulgar by a happy privilege of their ignorance are quite free from. They are afraid that a comet, by approaching a little too near the earth, may in an instant reduce us to ashes; or, that the sun one day or other will swallow us up; or, that this immense source of light and heat will at length be exhausted and leave us involved in a profound and eternal night. May not your fears, Madam, be said a little to resemble those of the Laputian school?

As to the *flapper*, answered she, I have nothing to do with that, especially when I am with you. But do you not think that there is some reason for me to be frighted at the terrible threatening of a perpetual night? Ought you not rather to think yourself obliged to me for interesting myself so much in the cause of *light*, which you have made your heroine? It would be quite shameful that I should shew more regard and concern for it, than yourself. You shall see, Madam, answered I, that these atomists have taken care to secure your repose, and preserve what you shew such a regard for. They will find you a method to recruit the sun with that facility which a philosopher is master of, who knows how to make all nature subservient to his schemes. They will make the seeds of light and heat, which are diffused through the universe, continually return back again into the sun, in order to repair his losses. They will place something round him with which he is sustained and restored just as a lamp is fed by oil or some other matter. We will call certain systems to our assistance which will lend us comets that from time to time shall fall into the sun and yield him fresh supplies: and if this be not sufficient, we will have recourse to some philosopher, who may find means to make a star fall into him. And if you have not confidence enough in human systems, we will call a celestial one to our aid, revealed to Adam by an angel in Milton, who assures us, that the sun draws his aliment from humid exhalations, and in a regular manner takes his supper every night with the ocean. Will you have any more? No, no, said she, the one half of thefe things is fufficient to diffipate the fears of a Laputian himfelf. And I hope there will be no need at prefent to trouble any philofopher; much lefs a fuperior Being.

I wifh, anfwered I, that your fears may never extend to any thing farther than philofophy, and that your beauty, as it has many other qualities in common with the fun, may have a common duration with him. But I am extremely glad that fince I have delivered you an opinion which at firft fight gave occafion to your fear, it is capable too of diffipating that fear: as you are fo very fubject to be frighted at every trifle, I do not know what would have happened, if I had told you the opinion of a famous antient, who affirmed the fun to be a mirror formed of a fubftance refembling the moft polifhed chryftal, that fends and reflects the light to us, which is tranfmitted to all parts of the univerfe, and there unites. What hopes fhould we have of finding proper materials above, to repolifh this mirror, if it fhould ever happen to be fullied and grow dim? Let him, replied the Marchionefs, who made the fun a mirror, contrive how to repolifh it when it fhall want it, I had rather imagine it to be the foul of the world, and to be itfelf the fource of light. You fhould have added, that it is the fource of colours too, anfwered I, fince without light thefe entirely vanifh and are no more. Say rather, replied the Marchionefs, that they are no longer vifible. Will you tell me that an hour after fun-fet, there are no colours in this picture? I fhould be glad to hear you prove to me that the picture too is vanifhed for the fame reafon, becaufe it is no longer vifible. The picture, anfwered I, and the canvas ftill remain, and upon it certain difpofitions in the figure and texture of thofe atoms, alks that are made use of in the painting

And these dispositions, at the approach
again make the colours mezzotintos and
, appear upon the canvas, and restore to
mmanding beauty, a flight of pillars, a ver-
or the opening blushes of the morning.
ll these objects vanish, as they are the re-
ination of those dispositions and light to-
ght allege the authority of Virgil upon this
informs us, that objects lose their colours
h of night. Lucretius*, who, in the most
has given us a body of this atomic philoso-
apprehend most terrible consequences from
that bodies and their principles are endued
For, says he,

lourless without a dye.
cannot to seeds agree;
t immortal all and free
and therefor things may fall to nought.

CREECH.

e consequences and verses, said the Marchi-
want evidence and explications. Descartes,
ill afford you enough of this, who has dif-
tter much more fully than Lucretius. His
different, but in this point he agrees with
But you want systems, and I must satisfy
see the most daring products of imagination,
or some time deceived those, who assumed
title of searchers after truth. The illusion
anished, and philosophers are grown more

* Proinde colore cave, &c.   Lucret.
D

cautious and difficult, and examine one another with [no more]
violence than the Egyptians did their dead before [they]
would allow them the honour of sepulture. Come, [explain]
the Marchioness, explain me this system of Descartes; [it]
shall not be so difficult as not to receive pleasure from [it],
even if it be such a one as you make me expect. It is [possible,]
Madam, answered I, but that every thing should [for]
this time be proposed to you under the form of a phil[oso]phical system.

Suppose to yourself, that all the matter, of which [the]
whole world is composed, was from the beginning divi[ded]
into exceeding small and equal particles, of a figure ne[arly]
resembling a dye. Suppose too, that some of these [par]ticles turn round one point, and some another, and [that]
at the same time they all turn round themselves lik[e a]
wheel, which, while it is moving to any particular s[pot,]
makes many revolutions about its self. The points ab[out]
which these particles turn are the stars, the most lumin[ous]
and shining points in the universe, and which will h[elp]
you to conceive it full of *vortices*, for this is the name t[hat]
is given to any mass of matter that is whirled round a p[oint]
or common centre, just like the circles of water in a ri[ver]
or the dust that flies when it is agitated by the wind. [I]
believe you will not scruple to grant the sun a *vortex* of [his]
own upon my assertion, since he is not at all inferior [to]
any of the stars. If you desire it, answered the Marc[hi]oness, I will go farther, and allow him the largest [and]
most magnificent *vortex* in the world. For I think [he]
highly deserves it, to whom we have so many obligatio[ns.]
Philosophy, answered I, is less interested, and has no m[ore]
partiality for the sun, than for the least star in the mi[lky]
way. It is sufficient if you grant the sun a *vortex*, b[ut]

[as] it will. From this *vortex*, you shall see the sun him[self] [a]rise; for hitherto I have supposed him and the stars [ex]ist, the better to assist your imagination; and with [the] sun, all the charms of *light* and *colour*, and I know [not] what besides. In short, it is like an inchanted palace, [whe]re you have only need to ask what you want, and it [will] appear in an instant.

What I have granted you is so little, replied the Mar[chi]oness, that I cannot flatter myself with the hopes of so [gre]at a happiness as you flatter me. The mathematicians, [ans]wered I, are said to resemble lovers. If what you [gra]nt them at first be ever so little, they know how to [ma]ke so good an advantage of it, as to lead you insensibly [fur]ther than you ever imagined. Now you are to consider [tha]t this philosopher, to whom you have granted what [you] think so slight a concession, was a mathematician. I [ha]ve as little skill in the artifices of love, said the Marchi[one]ss, as in those of philosophy and mathematics. But it [is i]nconceivable to me that any thing reasonable can be [pro]duced by these *vortices*, which after all are nothing [bu]t collections of extremely small particles, that keep whirl[ing] round a point at the same time that each of them turns [rou]nd itself. They may whirl on for ever, and I believe [tha]t will be the chief of their business. Who would ever [ha]ve imagined, answered I, that the accidental meeting [of] a hero and heroine in a romance, and a certain *Je ne [sç]ai quoi*, that he discovers in her, could have supplied [ma]tter for twenty volumes? and yet there are many in[sta]nces of this, perhaps too many, in a nation very near [ou]r own. And without giving the heroes any trouble in [thi]s affair; what an infinite number of things might there [be] produced from that *Je ne sçai quoi*, that every one sees

D 2

in you?——Let us see at present, said the marchioness, what Descartes' *vortices* will produce; for after these twenty volumes, I shall begin to think every thing possible.

These particles then, continued I, in the figure of a dye, which you now begin to have a better opinion of, whirling in this manner round themselves, must make terrible collisions, and, consequently, break the angles or points of each; which deprive them of a power of turning freely round themselves. You know, Madam, that, if any thing be taken away from the corners of a dye, it will grow round, and in proportion as the angles of what remains of the dye keep successively diminishing, it will gradually approach still nearer to the shape of a ball. And this you are to believe was the case with these particles, which by continually striking against one another, were at length changed from their first figure of a dye, to that of so many little balls or globules. The matter which arose from the shavings of these angles, and which by its continual collision must necessarily be reduced into very small and volatile particles, did not remain idle, but had its proper office. It immediately declared open war against the vacuum of the atomists, and threatened to destroy and banish it from the universe, wherever it was to be found. The first undertaking of this matter was to fill up those little voids which otherwise would have remained between the globules; for though they touched one another, yet there must have been some empty spaces between them arising from the nature of a globular figure. But without the assistance of this *matter*, there would have remained a much more considerable void in the centre of the *vortex*. The globules were reduced to a much smaller size than they were at first; and were proportionably removed from the centre, by a law common to all bodies moving in a circle; which recide as far as they possibly can from that point about which they turn. This matter then run into the midst of the *vortex* in order to fill the centre of it, and began itself to turn round together with the globules, and animate the rest of the *vortex*. This subtile and volatile substance, which is called the *matter of the first element*, or the *subtile matter*, forms nothing less than the sun and stars in the centre of the *vortices*; as the globules that turn round them, and which are called the *matter of the second element*, furnish matter for the heavens; and though the CARTESIANS have deprived it of that transparency and adamantine solidity that formerly rendered it so venerable among the antients, they have taken care however to atone for this injury, by making it the original of light, and by this means it has gained more than it lost.

What, cried the marchioness, are we got already to the origin of light? Your heroes and their twenty volumes have made a very bad use of their time, compared with us. If you give a farther attention, answered I, you will find they have made a much worse use of it, even than you believe. The system of Des Cartes presents you a scene, such as, I believe, you never beheld in the finest and most splended opera. The whole extent of the universe is sown and filled with innumerable *vortices* joined to one another of different size and figure, but all of them nearly round. These keep each other in a mutual equilibrium by their reciprocal pressure. In the midst of every one of these *vortices* is a star or a sun, that is to say, a large ball of *subtile matter* that strives to dilate itself, and presses the *vortex* all round. This pressure of the *subtile* communicated to the *globular matter*, or that of the second element, gives birth to *light* according to the opinion of Des Cartes. The different bigness of the star, and much more its distance from us, cause the light of it to appear more or less lively to our sight: and hence it is that the splendor of the sun in whose *vortex* we are

—— *with superior blaze*
Dims the pale lustre of the starry rays.

It is believed that Syrius, though his distance from us be more than two millions of millions of English miles, according to the calculation of a celebrated mathematician, is yet the nearest star that we have; because it appears larger than any of the rest, and its lively and sparkling light makes the longest resistance against the dazling splendor of the sun.

I suppose, said the Marchioness, that out of partiality to your Syrius, you omit that star which the peasants call Diana, and the poets the harbinger of the rising day, and to whom, comparing earthly with heavenly things, they give the same honours as to Aurora. You must take care, answered I, not to confound two things together, which are very different from each other, as a body that is luminous in itself, and one that derives all its splendor from another; or in other words, a sun and a planet. It is true, that all the planets, as Venus, which in the language of astronomy is the same as your Diana, Mercury, Mars, Jupiter, Saturn, and our earth itself, were antiently so many suns, and may, perhaps, for who can penetrate into the secrets of futurity? hereafter be again restored to that honour. I have not yet mentioned to you another species of matter which is called the *matter of the third element,* and which has occasioned the greatest and most remarkable revolutions that are left upon record in the annals of the Cartesian philosophy. Among the particles of that *subtile matter* of which the sun is composed, there are some that by their rugged and irregular figure unite and cling together, and by these means form masses that are sometimes bigger than our earth. These masses are driven away from the sun, and repelled to his superficies. The pressure that communicates itself from the *subtile* to the *globular matter*, or in other words, the *light* is interrupted in that part of the sun's superficies where these masses are placed, and from hence they appear to us as spots, which, turning round with the sun, eclipse part of his splendor and glory. Flattery perhaps made certain courtly astronomers take these spots for little planets, that get betwixt the sun and us, and made use of them to transport the families of those princes to heaven, from whom they expected some little pension on earth in exchange for the investiture of a thousand planets which they with great confidence promised them. Philosophical politeness transformed these masses into patches upon the sun's face; if you are better pleased with the idea under which they were represented to the queen of Prussia by the famous Mr. Leibnitz, who thought that philosophical terms should be softened for the ear of queens. The thing is too serious to bear a jest, said the Marchioness; patches as big as the earth might quite demolish a face.

Hitherto, continued I, our sun has been lucky enough to escape this misfortune. The motion and agitation of the subtile matter breaks and dissipates these masses as fast as they are formed. There once appeared one of these spots, which darkened the fifth part of the sun's disk. This was a most enormous and terrible bigness, enough to make astronomers tremble, and the whole world melancholy. The sun at last disengaged himself, and got the better of it, so there is now no reason to fear any such unlucky accident; but all the other funs were not born under such favourable circumstances. There are certain stars which are confiderably diminished, so that what has formerly been placed by astronomers among those of the second magnitude, is now scarce worthy of being reckoned among those of the sixth. This must be ascribed to these spots which by length of time are so increased, as to form a sort of crust almost over the whole star, and consequently weaken its light.

On the other hand, said the Marchioness, might not certain stars arrive to a greater magnitude, if the agitation of the *subtile matter* was strong enough to dissipate part of their crust? You are throughly possessed, Madam, answered I, with the spirit of Cartesianism: this sect places its glory in conjectures, and you have made a very good one. But what a terrible desolation would it make in the poor star, if this crust should entirely cover it, as it too often happens, and should be strong enough to resist the force of the *subtile matter* that strives to break and dissipate it! When this is the case, we may bid farewel to the sun or star which has lost that place of honour which it before held in the universe. Its light is suffocated by the crust, and from a luminous and splendid body, it becomes dark and cold. The force of its *vortex* is confiderably weakened as it arose from the *subtile matter*, which has now no communication with the globule. The *equilibrium* is broke, and consequently its *vortex* destroyed. Some one of the neighbouring stars carries it away with it, and now become a planet, it is forced to whirl round at the mercy of the most powerful. These are the most remarkable metamorphoses that can possibly happen, and to which our metaphorical suns here below are no less subject. When these begin to lose their lustre and have nothing left to feed that paſſion which ſo agreeably flatters the pride of the fair ſex, and which ought to be the ſubject of your philoſophy, they are carried away and become ſlaves to another, which for their conſolation they call virtue. Our fallen ſuns, anſwered ſhe, have at leaſt the advantage in this, that they acquire a fine name, and under the ſhelter of that they with great authority condemn what is no longer in their power to practiſe, and in ſome meaſure recover their loſt empire. But what conſolation is there for a miſerable ſun above, when it is inveloped with a cruſt, and changed to a planet? The conſolation, anſwered I, of not having an odious and imaginary empire after having been poſſeſſed of an amiable and real one; the conſolation, in ſhort, of not growing like an old *Sybile* after having reſembled one.

This miſerable metamorphoſis of a ſun to a planet, accompanied however with ſome degree of conſolation, is probably what happened to a fine ſtar which we have entirely loſt in the conſtellation of Caſſiopeia; and this too, according to the Carteſian ſyſtem, was the fate of our earth, which was once empreſs of an extenſive *vortex* crowned with light, and one of the brighteſt eyes of heaven; but at length inveloped with a deformed cruſt, unhappily loſt its power and ſplendor, and was carried away by the immenſe *vortex* of the ſun, as a ſtraw in a river by the impetuoſity of a whirlpool. In the ſame manner, the other planets that revolve about him, Jupiter, Saturn, Mercury, Mars, Venus, fell victims to his ſuperior power; nor could even the comets eſcape, though theſe are planets of a peculiar nature which keep rambling from one *vortex* to another, and like certain people among us here below, rove from one country and government to another. And theſe *vortices* are the grand machine invented chiefly by Des Cartes, to guide the planetary dance round the sun.

Is the earth then, replied the Marchioness, after a short pause, like the other planets obliged to dance round the sun? And do all the mighty preparations, you made with *your matter of the third element*, amount only to this? The earth, answered I, does not need that concern which you shew for her degradation from a sun to the inferior rank of a planet; since by this means she was destined to give birth to you, who are but another name for the most charming thing, that all the *vortices* of the universe put together could ever have produced. Is not this a sufficient compensation for her loss? If it was in the power of gallantry, answered the Marchioness, to make her amends, yours would certainly do it. But what can ever free her from the disgrace of being obliged among the croud of other planets to whirl round the sun like a straw, agitated by the caprice of a whirl-pool? I am sensible that you philosophers look upon the earth with great indifference, and suffer it to turn round without regret; but for my part— Let it whirl round for this time, answered I, upon the word of Des Cartes. Hereafter if you have a mind to be convinced with pleasure, we will read M. Fontenelle's dialogues upon the plurality of worlds. There you will see a Marchioness, who exactly resembles you in every accomplishment of mind, and whom you have nothing to envy but her philosopher. At present you are to look upon the earth only as a composition of the matter *of the third element*, which renders it opaque, and as a body which no longer shines by its own light; and by this means I believe you will be pretty indifferent towards it. A gloworm, one of those reptiles that glitter by night in the country, is much more worthy your attention; whatever is not luminous is nothing to us.

You have seen, continued I, what sort of a thing light is: you see too how the sun may continually supply so great a quantity of light as he does, without any expence to himself, which is what gave you such terrible apprehensions in the atomic system. He has nothing to do but to press the globular matter, and this pressure costs him nothing of his own, and since it is communicated on all sides, we are to conclude that he is luminous quite round. The light, according to Des Cartes, is but a moment in progress from the sun to us notwithstanding the distance of a million of miles. The globules of the second element are continued from the sun to the earth, like so many strings of beads, and touch one another. In the instant that the first in the string moves, or endeavours to move, it must also endeavour to move the last. Just as a pole, though ever so long, in the moment that one end moves, the other moves also.

The meaning of all this is, answered the Marchioness, that by means of these *vortices* philosophers may make and give a reason for every thing. In a moment's time we have produced the sun, stars, planets, comets, the earth and light. I suppose we shall form colours with the same facility. Nothing more easy to Des Cartes, I replied. As motion or a tendency to motion in the celestial matter, raises in us the sensation of light, so the different motions of this matter excite in us the perception of different colours, which are nothing but certain modes in which bodies receive light, and afterwards transmit it to our eye. These modes consist in the increase or diminution of that motion, by which the globules of light naturally turn round themselves, and which is called the motion of rotation. Thus those bodies, whose superficies is disposed in such a manner as considerably to augment this motion of rotation in the globules of light which fall upon them, and are thence transmitted to us, appear to our sight red; those which increase the motion somewhat less, appear yellow: those, which considerably diminish it, appear blue, and those which diminish it in such a manner that these globules turn round slower than usual, appear green; and to conclude, those bodies, that transmit a great number of globules of light without altering their motion, appear to us white, and those seem black, which extinguish them, and as it were absorb the light. Here then you have the origin of colours, do you desire any thing more? It is only speaking; the *vortices* are as useful to Des Cartes as the cocao-tree to the Indians, which supplies them with all they want.

No, no, said the Marchioness, let us at present confine ourselves to colours: I need only increase or diminish the motion of rotation, in the globules of light, in order to form the shades of a fine silk, and variegate the parterre of a garden with the different beauties of hyacinths, anemonies and violets, in short, to diversify the face of nature just as I please. Rather, said I, if this increase or diminution should give you any trouble, you need only suppose the globules of light to be entirely deprived of all rotation, which we will grant them only in the very action of variegating your silk or parterre, or in other words, in being repelled from the bodies upon which they fall. You may freely choose which of these methods suits you best. Each of them will equally serve your purpose. Des Cartes, seems to have had this too in common with the phy-

e thought it unworthy his fruitful imagina-
himself to one single method of making his
l. Notwithstanding your malicious insinua-
he Marchioness, I think myself much obliged
for this copiousness. I dare say it will not
plaining how it comes to pass that one body
ie globules of light a certain rotation, and
a different one. You are not confined here
ered I, but have free liberty of choosing what
ike best for the explanation of the thing in
r different figures of those particles of which
of bodies are composed; or their different
heir different inclination towards each other,
more or less smooth, and a thousand other
ou may imagine to yourself. By these means
rous philosopher compose not only the finery
the variegated beauties of a garden, but all
of a Paul Veronese or the delicacy of Titian;
arises that lively bloom on your complexion,
is not all the art of Paul and Titian could
tated. I should not have thought, answered
colouring of my cheeks would ever have en-
e Cartesian system. It enters, answered I,
stems more generally understood, and of
re importance than those of philosophy. But
ist receive great honour from the explication
l a phenomenon.
said the Marchioness, that this great plenty
I above all the simplicity that reigns through-
n, quite charms me, not to say any thing of
ies which it removes in all the rest. I should
: how any other woman in my place would
E

guard against it. I am too well acquainted with the language of ladies, answered I, not to believe you already conquered. You have not sufficiently closed your ears to the song of this philosophical syren, nor guarded your heart against the alluring pleasures in the luxurious garden of this Cartesian enchantress. But you have forgot that yourself at first condemned this precipitation in building systems, which cannot afterwards bear up against the obstinacy of observators. Hypotheses, or imaginary systems cannot long resist the force of experiments, which are justly called by a man, who carried them farther than perhaps any one that may follow him, natural revelations. A liar, even if he was as ingenious as he in Corneille's comedy, will at last be found out. I had no notion, said she, that so many things could have been produced from so little a matter, as these whirling particles, and I think upon this account a little precipitation might be excused, and all this moralizing laid aside. I am extremely fond of the Chinese, because I am told they effect whatever they take in hand, with much fewer instruments and less apparatus than we do. And I think French music much preferable to ours, because by a few simple and plain notes it touches the heart, and moves the passions. Whereas ours, with all its divisions, fugues and shakes, leaves us for the most part in a tedious and stupid tranquillity. Those, who for every little thing make use of such great machines, put me in mind of the dictators antiently elected at Rome, with the utmost solemnity, and who never omitted choosing a master of horse for no other end, than to fix a nail in the capitol. You may add, said I, since you seek for examples illustriously ridiculous, those kings of Persia, who never eat, walk, or go into the seraglio, till an astro-

many obfervations and calculations, has af-
hat it is a lucky time to undertake one or
important enterprizes. If we had been in
many aftrologers, how many calculations,
ave been employed before you could have
philofopher! which I take to be a thing of
importance, than the walk of a king. I am
ered fhe, that before the aftrologer had fi-
alculations, my inclination for philofophy
left me. But thanks to my good fortune,
rn in a country, where if we have a mind to
philofophical difcourfes, we may do either
g the ftars or the fky any trouble about it.
ather to thank your good fortune, Madam,
or being born in a country where your charms
hofe of the eaftern beauties, confined to the
s of a feraglio.
e reflections of yours, faid the Marchionefs,
e me lofe fight of our colours, whofe variety
he more, becaufe the production of them coft
rouble. But how fhall we produce thofe va-
which appear in looking through a certain
once faw placed over-againft a window? per-
re fome other fort of motion to produce thefe
h only appear to be in objects, when they
pon through one of thefe glaffes. You may
anfwered I, in the very fame manner as the
eed only make the globules of light that pafs
glafs you mentioned, which is called a *prifm*,
according to thofe rules you have already
according as the variety of colours which it
uire. As to that diftinction, which you feem

to put upon those colours which are really in bodies, and those which are so only in appearance, Des Cartes will not grant it you; for he, as well as the atomists, as you may remember, asserts, that there are absolutely no colours in bodies, and that they only appear to be so. Thus for instance, betwixt the red on your cheeks, and that in the rainbow, or *prism*, there is no sort of difference, only perhaps it would be more pleasant to make observations on one than the other. But after all, they are of the same nature, and only apparent. Do you think, continued I laughing, that so many poets would have compared fine ladies to the rainbow, if there had not been some resemblance in their colour? as, for example, one of the greatest philosophers in our time has done in those sublime verses, where he is describing some beauty who perhaps resembled you.

> * *Tale in somma ne gia qual di rubini*
> *E d'or ricca, e di gemme e d'ostro adorno*
> *Sorger veggiam la matutina aurora.*
> *O qual sul variato e lucid arco*
> *Apparir suol dopo nembosa pioggia*
> *Di taumante la figlia; allorchè, i venti venti*
> *Si stan sospesi a vagheggiarla e intanto*
> *L' insano mar depon l' ira, e s'achera.*

You see, said I, that one of the most splended and pompous similes, that the poets have in their whole collection, would have been guilty of too essential an error.

Seriously, answered the Marchioness, I always thought that the colour on my cheeks, whatever it be, was really

---

* As our author does not mention where he had these verses, I would not venture to translate them from the Italian, since I am not certain, whether they were not originally written in English.

here, and that the prism or the rainbow were only in appearance; pray explain this paradox to me, which, to say truth, I am very much perplexed with; and deliver me from the uneasiness I cannot help feeling on your comparing me to the rainbow, notwithstanding you made me a great compliment by this fine simile. This, said I, is reducing things to that simplicity you seemed so fond of, by taking away the distinction which you put between real and apparent colours. But the interest you have in this distinction, and your self-love, that makes you tremble at the thoughts of losing your roses and lilies, to speak in the pastoral style, has at present got the better of your love of simplicity. I will engage there are many ladies who would have the same scruples: but after all, you cannot with honour adopt a system without being willing to admit the consequences. We have before said, that there is in bodies only a certain disposition and texture of parts, and in the globules of light a certain rotation which these parts give them. These globules in a certain manner tickling and shaking the nerves of the *retina*, which is a very thin membrane at the bottom of the eye, give us the idea of some colour, which we by the help of our imagination refer to the body from whence those globules of light are derived to us. But I think we are called to dinner, and it is time for us to see what taste our imagination will help us to give the soup. Our imagination, replied the Marchioness! I do not know whether he, who has laboured these three hours to give it a real taste, will be very well pleased with you philosophical gentlemen, who would reduce every thing to mere appearance. I dare say, answered I, that he will give himself very little trouble about such a trifle as a philoso-

phical opinion. But however, if he did, he muſt bear i[t]
for as bodies are in reality without colour, ſo they a[re]
likewiſe without taſte, ſmell, ſound, heat, cold, and ev[en]
when they appear moſt luminous, without light.

The Marchioneſs was very deſirous that I ſhould expla[in]
this paradox more fully: but I aſſured her, that if [we]
ſtayed till the ſoup wanted heating again, not the fine[ſt]
and moſt ſimple explications in the world would help o[ur]
imagination to give it a good taſte. She was fully co[n]
vinced of this truth, and we ended our diſcourſe in t[he]
manner of Homer's gods, who after their conſultatio[n]
are ſure never to forget their ambroſia.

DIALOGUE II.

That qualities, such as light, colours, and the like, are not really in bodies. Metaphysical doubts concerning our sensations of them. Explication of the general principles of optics.

ALL the while we were at dinner, the Marchioness entertained herself with making the globules of light turn round, sometimes one way, sometimes another, as the different colours of the objects before us required, and looked upon herself, as she said, to be the empress and arbitratress of nature, since she was possessed of materials to diversify it as many ways as she pleased. As soon as dinner was over, and we had returned into the garden, I am ready, said she, to deprive the soup of all taste, and willingly renounce every colour, even what I had the greatest fondness for. In short, I will be quite a Cartesian, provided you can furnish me with good reasons. These globules, it is true, lead me to strange consequences, but perhaps they may furnish me with some expedient to evade them. You treat philosophy, answered I, as attorneys do the law. But there is no expedient that will hold good at the severe tribunal of reason. Not all the monarchs in the universe, nor all the beauties which are far more powerful, can influence the impartial judgment of philosophy, nor induce it to interpret the least text in their favour. This is a trial, a mortification that Des Cartes will make you undergo in your noviciate of philosophy. But are you terrified at so small a hardship as this? Take courage and fear nothing; you will at last add to the pleasure you receive from your senses, that of contending with them, and giving them no credit.

Hitherto, said the Marchioness, I have only the mortification of seeing that we are under a perpetual delusion, since, if what you say be true, things appear to us very different from what they really are. Bodies appear to us of a certain colour, whereas there is really nothing else in them but a certain disposition of parts. They seem to us to be hot, cold, and yet they are possessed of none of these qualities. Really I cannot help thinking, that we are in a very strange condition. It is certainly very strange, answered I. Our knowlege can make but very little progress, unless it be conducted by the senses. They continually make us believe things, which a more refined sense, or our reason, afterwards contradicts. You think, for instance, that your hands, which have been the subject of so many fine verses, are smooth and polished; and possibly might be greatly offended, if any one should dare to dispute them this quality. And yet if you were to look upon them through a microscope, you would be surprized to see a great number of pores that separate the texture of them, and to find that they are covered with scales like those of a fish. You would discover in them cavities, promontories; vallies and hills, for the abode of a nation of little animals, who perhaps spend their life there. And to increase your wonder, you would be presented with the sight of rivers and seas. In short you would not know them again, and you would be obliged to confess that they are very different from those which your poets describe. Nature, said the Marchioness, has done us a great favour in not making our senses too refined. It would be very bad for us, if our touch was exquisite enough to feel all that the microscope discovers to our sight. We should certainly be extremely unhappy, answered I, if our sensations were so perfect, that in handling the smoothest surface, our touch should fail us at every pore, and every little eminence should make us shudder. It is to the silence of our reason, and the want of more refined senses, that we owe our perceptions of pleasure. And he gave a very just definition of our happiness, who affirmed, that the most tranquil possession of pleasure consists in our being agreeably deceived.

It must be confessed, replied the Marchioness, that our sex is greatly obliged to the complaisance of philosophers, who, notwithstanding they are so well acquainted with the nature of our superficies, are so genteel as to behave towards us like the rest of mankind. But if I had a mind to please any ignorant person, the very first thing I would do, should be to forbid him the holding any correspondence with those gentlemen who deal in microscopes; for these might do me a very great prejudice. Not all the microscopes nor all the philosophy in the world, answered I, could ever hinder your appearing agreeable to the naked eye, and even a Cleopatra might be contented with this. Virgil makes Corydon warn his Alexis not to confide in his beauteous colour. But I may freely give you leave to confide in your hands.

As our senses are not microscopical, so neither are our hearts philosophical. It would be very bad for us, if our pleasure was in the hands of philosophers, and if beauty, in order to prove its existence, must stand out against all the experiments of a naturalist. This is just as if the chastity of a lady should depend upon the ill-grounded suspicion, and diligent enquiry of a jealous husband. These two kinds of men have this in common, that they both equally tend to destroy the most valuable things in the world.

But philosophers, said the Marchioness, destroy without mercy; for they can leave but very little else to bodies, after they have deprived them of colour, taste, and those many other qualities which they have taken from them. They leave them, answered I, in possession of extension, that is, length, breadth, and depth; impenetrability, motion, figure, and all the fine things that mathematicians and mechanics deduce from these qualities, upon which I could produce you so many formidable volumes, that all which has been written upon the *Crusca*, would seem, compared to these, no more than a king's declaration of love. Do not you think it enough for bodies that they are no more than bodies? Besides, what philosophers do with regard to those qualities we were speaking of, is not properly a destruction: they take nothing away from bodies, but what was falsely applied to them, and what they had unjustly possessed; and restore those qualities to us, to whom they rightly and properly belong. Prescription has at present no influence on philosophy, as it formerly had. If a lover, for example, should say, that there was hope in a certain favourable glance, which had darted on him through a fan, what harm would a philosopher do, who, without destroying either the hope or the glance, should tell him that there was nothing in the glance, but a particular motion of the eye, caused by certain muscles, either from a principle of pity, or if we would trace the thing to its original, coquetry: but that the hope was entirely of himself, and excited by the means of that n the same manner, when we are pricked the pain is entirely in ourselves; and there he needle but a motion by which it disjoins the fibres of our body: this separation is we feel pain. In short, bodies are only nsequently can have no properties but what ltter; and these the Cartesians have conion, mutual impenetrability, diversity of different disposition of parts. And these to give bodies a power of exciting difus, as those of light, colours, taste, and the necessary, for instance, that colour should the surface of a body, in order to make me r, any more than it is necessary for pain to , in order to make me feel it when I am sufficient that as the needle causes a certain ιe fibres of my body, by the means of which ι, so that particular rotation, which is in ed from the surface of a body, should cause ι upon the nerves of the retina, which care to the brain excites in me the idea, or, as e sensation of colour. Thus, if in any body ain motion by which it pressed the globules lement, and these globules be carried to our raise in us the idea of light. A certain conarticles, or perhaps certain little animals ιodies, by playing upon the nerves of the a particular manner, raise in us the sensaιste. These sensations are generally raised ι of certain bodies, and because we see neiicles nor the little animals which are in bules of the second element, nor the imis made upon our nerves, we ascribe to those bodies both light, colours and taste, which in reality are only in ourselves. Reason at length convinces us of the illusion that our imagination continually puts upon us, and assures us, that the delightful and hitherto undefined taste of the pine-apple, the pleasing verdure of a meadow, and even the light of the sun which animates and revives the whole universe, are all our own.

I understand you, said the Marchioness; we are enriched at another's expence, and are like antient Rome, which founded its grandeur upon the spoils of the whole universe. Philosophy would be in a bad state, answered I, if its rights had no better foundation, than those of policy and ambition. I see you have not yet a right notion of it. In order to convince yourself that philosophy is no usurper, but only takes its due, press one corner of your eye with your finger, and you will see on the opposite part a round flame of a reddish colour. In this case there is certainly neither light nor colour without your eye. The only reason of your seeing them is the pressure which your finger makes upon the nerves of your eye. The globules of light, which flow from the surfaces of bodies, occasion the same effect upon the eye as your finger, only their operation is more imperceptible. The different disposition and configuration of the parts of a body, are the reason why the globules make different impressions upon us. The power of a body's exciting in us the idea of any particular colour, consists alone in this disposition, and the configuration of its parts. Is it not evident from hence, that if this disposition be changed, the colour is changed also? which could not happen if the colour was really in the parts of the body itself. Coral, which is of a fine red, if it be ground to powder turns pale. One liquid mixed with another changes its colour. The reason of all this

, that the disposition and configuration of the parts of these bodies are changed by being ground or mixt, and from hence they transmit the light to us in a different manner, and consequently our idea of the colour is changed; from no other reason proceed the venerable white locks of old age; the transient whiteness of many animals of the north in winter. From hence too it is, that certain roses in China are in the same day both white and purple. From this cause arises that surprising variation of colour which generally follows the change of passions in the camelion, which has furnished the moralists and poets with so many allusions, the antients with so many fables, and the moderns with so many observations. And what is it else but one disposition which hinders us from seeing you goddesses when you first rise, and another which gives you to our sight and adorations after you have spent two or three hours in the sacred rites of the toilet?

I perceive, replied the Marchioness, that there is nothing secret to philosophy; we may hide ourselves from men, but not from philosophers. And indeed to what purpose would it be for us to endeavour to conceal ourselves from a set of people who are quick sighted enough to discover the globules of light endowed with a certain motion, and those nerves and fibres to which this motion is communicated and thence conveyed to the brain? A sight which mortal eyes have never yet penetrated into. But I must confess, I stand in need of your assistance to guide me through this obscure labyrinth. I do not see what relation all these motions have to any colour that I have a conception of. This is a thing which seems to me quite different from these motions. Have you any better conception, answered I, of the relation between the idea of pain, and a separa-

F

tion of the fibres of your hand? Or between the idea of hope and a certain motion in the muscles of an eye? And yet you see that these things are in fact connected, and that the one is the cause, or at least the occasion, of the other. You seek for more than it is possible to give you. Unhappily for us, those things which are of the greatest importance to human knowlege are the most doubtful. Who can tell you in what manner objects occasion certain ideas in the soul, and how the soul on the other hand gives certain motions to the body? how the soul which is unextended, yet is present in every part of our whole machine, and though incapable of being seen or felt, yet sees and feels every thing? Philosophers can with a great deal of ease transmit the motion of the globules of light, or any other motion, to the nerves, and from these to the brain, where they all terminate, either by means of a fluid that runs through them, or a certain tremor raised in them. Nay, philosophers will go yet farther, and transmit this motion to certain parts of the brain which are imagined to be the seat of the soul. But how these motions, when they are arrived to the brain or seat of the soul, should produce in it different ideas, is an absolute mystery. This passage, which in appearance is so short, is to philosophers what the innavigable ocean was to the antients. What communication, what connexion can there be between body and soul, between extension and thought, motion and idea, matter and spirit? What sort of communication these can have with one another, is beyond the reach of our imagination. The same, answered she smiling, that Æneas had with the shade of his father Anchises in the Elysian fields. They mutually communicate the most agreeable things in the world to one another, but when Æneas attempts to embrace the old man, he vanishes away and is dissipated into air.

We may draw a fine allegory from this passage, answered which would have done great honour to a learned and musty commentator of the last age. Now in order to put our allegory in a clear light, and to let you see on the other hand that nothing is able to discourage a set of people brought up and educated in the midst of difficulties, some of them will tell you, that there is a certain correspondence or pre-established harmony betwixt soul and body, so that though they have no more connexion with each other, than a harlequin dance in our operas has with the death of Dido, or the fate of Rome; yet by virtue of this pre-established harmony, at the same time that certain motions happen in the one, certain ideas and desires arise in the other. In short, that they are like two clocks independent of each other, whose weights are adjusted in such a manner, that when this strikes one, that shall always strike two, and so on. Your Des Cartes will tell you that upon occasion, when bodies without us in the material world excite certain motions in our body, the soul sees certain ideas in the intellectual world. So that in the material world, you have nothing but extension, and certain motions, and configurations, and whatever other qualities you possess, and which render you so agreeable and charming, exist only in the intellectual world. Others will tell you, that by means of certain motions in the body, God reveals and displays certain ideas to the soul. But they have so little regard for any connexion between these motions and our ideas, that they affirm, we might as well hear with our eyes, or see with our ears, provided the laws of the union of the soul and body were different from what they now are, which is not impossible, since these laws are merely arbitrary. One of the laws of this union is, that when there are certain motions impressed on one of the membranes of the eye, the idea of light should be raised in us, and in the same manner, when certain motions are made upon a membrane of the ear, we should perceive the idea of sound. And as these things are independent of one another, why might not the idea of light arise from certain motions upon the ear, and that of sound from certain motions impressed on the eye?

And why, said the marchioness, may we not rather suppose that there are some secret dependencies between these things, which your philosophers may not have been acquainted with? The vulgar hide their ignorance under the vail of obstinacy, and do not the learned endeavour to conceal theirs in doubts and questions? Your suspicion at least is reasonable, answered I. Our horizon is but faintly illuminated with the beams of a glimmering twilight, and we pretend to see as clearly as if it was full day. We continually act, especially with regard to metaphysics, as Columbus would have done, if he had pretended to write us a complete description of America, and given an account of its inhabitants, rivers and mountains, when he had only seen a little tract of this country, and did not know whether it was an island or a continent. We reason upon the chimeras of our own fancy, we destroy and build systems, we raise doubts, and think to resolve them without agreeing upon so much as their first ideas. One of the most elegant geniuses of England, who in our days has revived the polite court of Charles II. in that happy country, in a little, but very valuable piece, which he wrote against one of the most celebrated metaphysicians of

ur time, compares thofe gentlemen to fine riders in a
' manage, who fhow their addrefs and dexterity by mak-
' ing their horfe go backwards or fideways, and all ways,
' and at length after having laboured round and round
' for two or three hours, get down juft where they got up."
However it be with thefe metaphyfical jockies, it is certain,
that fome things produce others very different from them.
The Americans without doubt would be extremely furprized to hear that certain cyphers, as the letters of the
alphabet, could tranfmit the hiftory of a nation to pofterity,
and furnifh two people with means of communicating their
thoughts, quarrelling or making love at the diftance of
four thoufand miles, juft as well as if they were prefent
with each other. And would not the Chinefe be greatly
aftonifhed to fee that certain marks drawn upon lines fhould
produce founds, concords, and in fhort, a concert of
mufic?

As I imitate thefe in their furprize, replied the Marchionefs, I will imitate them too in their docility, which they
difcover in embracing whatever we teach them as reafonable even at the expence of their felf-love. We muft then
folemnly abjure all thofe charms which you call rofes and
lilies, and fubmit to that philofophy which deprives us
of them, perhaps to give us in exchange fome greater
good. I admire your moderation, anfwered I, in agreeing to this Cartefian philofophy, which, to fay truth, is
fomewhat injurious to fine ladies. When the philofophy
of Ariftotle was in vogue, who afferted that qualities were
really in bodies, the ladies might be fomething vainer of
their beauty. But now they muft renounce the very things
upon which that vanity was principally founded. It is
true, that with globules alone, a bare difpofition of parts,

you will still continue to make the same conquests as y[ou]
did before with the help of colour itself. But it is tr[ue]
on the other hand, that it is for ever gone without a[ny]
hopes of being recovered again. However, if you are a-
fraid that this system may do you any sort of injury, yo[u]
need only name the person whom you have a desire to pleas[e]
and I will promise you never to let him into the secrets o[f]
philosophy.

Till there appears another system to deprive us of tha[t]
disposition of parts which this leaves us, replied she, I d[o]
not see, that we have any thing to fear, since after all
one certain disposition has only one certain idea affixed to
it. So that the disposition, which excites the idea of a fine
red in you, cannot produce that of a yellow or brown in
another person. And thus I think we are secure. Seriously, answered I, I do not at all doubt that beauties are
secure in any system of philosophy whatever. But that a
certain disposition of the parts of a body should excite
the same idea in all men, is what I cannot assure you of.
Who can tell whether the leaves of these trees that I see
of one colour which I call green, may not appear to your
sight of another colour which I should call red or yellow,
or perhaps of some other colour, of which I have no idea?
You would render me too philosophical, said the Marchioness, and after this I shall be utterly at a loss how to converse with mankind. You have made me already rob bodies of light, colours, taste, smell, and every other quality
which these have never made any scruple to grant them,
and would be greatly offended at any attempt to take them
away. But not content with all this, you would have
me confess that a colour which appears green to some,
should seem to others red, yellow, or some other colour,

On LIGHT and COLOURS.

perhaps, of which I have no idea. Is it possible to offer a greater affront to mankind, than to contradict a thing they are so sensibly persuaded of, and assert that they do not all see colours in the same manner? I will venture to tell you still more, answered I, for to shew a regard to mankind, whom you seem so fearful of offending, in this point, is not possible for any one who has ever conversed with them. Who can tell whether these very trees, which I see of one certain height, may not appear to you of another? So that what I, for instance, call ten foot high, may appear to your eyes of a height which I should call eight, or twenty feet. You have a mind to divert yourself at my expence, said the Marchioness, interrupting me. We both agree in calling this tree so many foot high, as well as in calling the leaves green. How then can what you say be true? We agree, answered I, in words, but perhaps not in things. Two people, one of which should give a chief magistrate the name of king, from whose good or ill administration depend the life and properties of his subjects; and the other should give the name of king to a chief magistrate, who is only the ratifier and guardian of the laws of nature, to which he, as well as the rest, is subjected: these two people would both agree in the sound, by which they denote their chief magistrate, but not in the idea which they annex to this sound. Both you and I had a certain measure at first shewn us, which though it appears to you of a different size from what it does to me, yet both of us agree in calling it a foot, because we are told that mankind distinguished such a measure by that name. According to this, which is the rule of our mensurations, we both say that this tree is so many foot high, though it may appear to me of a greater or less height than it does to you, and so every other thing in proportion to the different idea we may possibly have of a foot. Who can tell then, but you may appear to yourself, and I to you, like one of Gulliver's Brobdingnagians; on the contrary each of us may appear to my sight as small as a Lilliputian does to yours, and who knows too but you may see the whole world after the proportion of my Brobdingnagian, and I of the same size as your Lilliputian; so that if it were possible for us to see with each other's eyes, which would be a good exchange for me, you would despise the diminutive size of my Colossuses, and I should tremble at the gigantic stature of your pigmies. We may easily transfer the same way of reasoning to colours. We here too agree upon names, but may very probably differ in things. Each of us, for instance, calls the leaves of this tree green, because we were at first told that the colour of leaves was green; but it is possible, that if things could appear to your eyes as they do to mine, you would be surprized to see these trees and the whole country clothed in a colour which you perhaps might call purple or some other. Because we see that all men resemble one another in the make of their body, when they have all two eyes, one mouth, two legs, and two hands, we are led to imagine from thence that they must all resemble each other in their ideas, and from hence arise many inconveniences in society which would not have happened, had men been a little more philosophical than they are. From hence it is, that a politician, when you are thinking on something quite different from his projects, will plague you with a long account of the end and intentions of all the privy councils in Europe, and the division which he has already made in Italy; for he thinks it impossible that a man, who resem-

es him in his outward appearance, should not equally
interest himself in his visionary schemes. From the same
cause a lover will talk you dead with the history of his
continual sighs and hopeless passion. In short, this mistaken notion gives birth to numberless other inconveniences
in society. None greater, said the Marchioness, than the
philosophers who endeavour to reverse the ideas that mankind have formed to themselves, and make us believe that
we do not all see the same thing of the same size and colour. Cannot you find some method to explain to me
whether the world really appears so different to different
persons, as you say it does?

It is not possible, answered I, to find such a method as
you require, unless there could be any one measure which
all men were certain of seeing absolutely of the same size,
and certain colours which, in the same manner, they could
be assured, appear the same to all eyes, and to these they
might refer all other colours, as well as all other sizes
to the measure. As those two people who make use of
the same word *king* to signify their chief magistrate, though
the one be in effect very different from the other, can never come to a clear explanation of the different ideas they
would annex to the same word, unless they define and
compare it with other words, and more simple ideas, such
as both parties are agreed upon. Now red, yellow, and
the smallest imaginable measure, are in themselves such
simple ideas, that they can neither be defined nor compared with other ideas more simple. Therefor we have
no way of knowing whether all men have the same conceptions of them, or not, so that mankind are much to
blame in being so confident that the world appears in the

same manner to all, for it is a great chance but they a mistaken in this affair.

But what ill consequences can there possibly follow fro our saying that the world appears to every single man di ferent from what it does to all the rest? Nay, if we shou go farther, and say that even the world itself does not e ist, and that all these bodies, this sun, these stars, an these fine ladies, are nothing else but dreams and appear ances. There is one philosopher who affirmed, that a person need only to have slept once in his life-time, to be convinced of this. So that while some are disputing about the manner in which the world exists, others absolutely deny that it exists at all. But though I have slept more than once in my life, I will not preach up a system to you which would mutually destroy us both. I will rather assure you, that though we really should see the world in different manners, yet I am willing for my own interest to consult your preservation. They will all agree in saying, that this tree is so many feet high, and the leaves green, and that you are of a just height and a fine complexion; and does not this difference of ideas diffuse an infinite variety over the whole system of nature, which seems even in the minutest things to take a pleasure in diversifying herself a thousand ways? but what a pleasure must you find in imagining yourself to appear to some under the height of a wax baby, and to others as tall as the image of Flora at Farnese! to some of an azure complexion, with the green locks of a Nereid, and to others of a vermilion dye, and adorned with the rosy tresses of Aurora, and under these different aspects, to be agreeable to all, and adored under various forms, as the goddesses formerly were among the antients. I must confess this imagination, that every sin-

On LIGHT and COLOURS. 73

e man sees the face of the world in a manner different
om all the rest, though, if you will have it so, it be a
oubtful point, gives me so much pleasure, that I make
o scruple of carrying it beyond size and colours, to taste,
nell, and all other qualities. I said, *if you will have it so,*
nly out of complaisance to you; for if it be considered
ow very different the nature of things is from what it
ppears to our sight, since we reckon, for instance, those
odies to be smooth and solid, which are in reality full of
ores, cavities, and risings, and imagine them to be en-
ued with colour, taste, and other qualities which exist
nly in ourselves: when we consider too that the same bo-
ies have a different appearance according to their distance
nd the other circumstances in which they are seen; when
ll this, I say, is well considered, I do not know whether
ve may not affirm that every single man sees them in a dif-
erent manner from all the rest, and that our judgment
s as much deceived in supposing that the same things raise
he same ideas in different persons, as it evidently is in the
ther respect; at least we may reasonably doubt whether
t be not so. You will say perhaps, that this is raising
loubts and questions to hide our ignorance. But it is how-
ver one of the parts of a philosopher to search for motives
pon which he may form rational doubts upon things, or
ather, such is our misfortune, this is the best part of phi-
osophy. However, we every day clearly see that the
ame objects do in effect appear differently to different per-
ons: not to say any thing of the more important affairs
of morality, law, and politics, where what is esteemed in
one nation an object of veneration and respect, is reckoned
candalous and detestable in another. Did not the ladies
n one age drive all the colour out of their cheeks, and

affect a pale languid look, which were capable of inspir-
ing the moſt lively ſentiments, at a time when a painted
face would have been as ſhocking as a fury. But in the
next age, this very fury becomes a Venus, and inſtead of
ſighs and fine ſpeeches, the pale beauties are recommended
to the care of a phyſician, or the uſe of Spaniſh wool.
Were not the very ſame graſhoppers, that weary us with
their troubleſome chirping, called by an ancient poet the
ſweet harbingers of the ſummer? There are whole nations
who eſteem black teeth a ſingular beauty, and others who
paint one eye white, and the other red or yellow. In
ſome other countries, a beau ſacrifices and gaſhes his face
to appear more agreeable to the eyes of a brutiſh creature,
who is alone the miſtreſs of his heart. An olive complexion joined to a long head, a pair of deep ſunk black eyes,
a flat noſe, and the feet of a baby, are charms that make
great havock in the hearts of the Chineſe, and occaſion
whole volumes of gallant verſes and love epiſtles. Our Galatea's and Venus's would not get ſo much as one *billet
doux*, or a ſingle ode there, but would be looked upon as
mere caricatures. In the ſame country, learning is a ſtep
to the higheſt honours of ſtate, and there is more ceremony
in making a doctor there, than the Polanders uſe in elect-
ing a king. Are not muſic and dancing, which are with
us, as antiently among the Greeks, an exerciſe for perſons
of the firſt rank, looked upon in Perſia, as they formerly
were at Rome, as ſcandalous employments? And would
not the ſame ladies, who cauſe ſo many commotions and
diſturbances in Europe, be cloſe confined in a ſeraglio and
guarded by eunuchs in the eaſtern countries? If you will
not conſent to admit a different appearance of things between men, yet you muſt allow it to be ſo with regard to

nſtance, between us and the orientals, un-
ept ſome particular follies which ſeem to
 more extenſive and univerſal right over
: antients Greeks, the Romans, Orientals
 though ſeparated from each other by ſuch
 id and ſo many ſeas, yet all agreed in the
 1, that when the moon was in an eclipſe,
 ined by the ſhadow of the earth, that de-
 ſun's light, ſhe was in great danger, and
 iely hard, and imagined they could be of
 y howling, rattling with their timbrels, and
 iſt horrible outcries and noiſes they could

 he Marchioneſs, you begin to grow a little
  after this philoſophical enthuſiaſm which
 1 ſo far, that you endeavoured to reverſe the
 f things. But you have now conſented to
 e think alike in theſe opinions which you
  As to all the reſt, I am very well ſatisfied,
 iis difference of ideas at ſo great a diſtance
 is and the Oriental countries.
  make you ſtill eaſier, anſwered I, we will
 e theſe different ways of conception at a dif-
 ter, and in proportion as you grow a greater
 ihiloſophy, we will bring them gradually
 till at laſt we will agree to put ſome differ-
 your ideas and mine, and from thence be-
 eyes of ſome perſons to whom the ſame ob-
 gger when ſeen through one eye, than it
 ked upon by the other.
  poſſible, ſaid the Marchioneſs? There is no
 iſionary fancies, and you ſeem reſolved to
      G

put me to the utmost proof of my credulity. Not contented to make a difference of ideas between different persons, you carry your notions so far as to make this difference between the two eyes of the same person. I must confess, I think this a very daring way of proceeding. Did not Gassendus, answered I, one of the celebrated philosophers of the last age, affirm that he saw the characters of a book larger through one of his eyes, than the other? You see the fault is not to be thrown upon me, but upon the eyes of Gassendus. You would find many other persons with these sort of eyes, if they were but as curious in examining their senses as they are diligent in making use of them. To some persons an object is said to appear green when looked at through one eye, and yellow or blue, when seen by the other. But do not we see every day, that what one person esteemeth cold, another calls hot? Or rather do not we ourselves think the same thing to be cold or hot, according to our different dispositions? Would not the very same thing that Milo might have thought smooth as a mirror, appear rough as a nettle to that luxurious youth whose bed was strowed with roses, and who could not sleep for a whole night, because a single leaf happened to be doubled? And do not these different sensations which are so extremely opposite, as hot and cold, smooth and rough, proceed from a different disposition of the sensitive organs; from a different affection of the nerves, or the more or less delicate texture of the parts appointed to carry these sensations to the brain? and is it not very probable too, that these differences may be in that membrane of the eye, upon which the images of objects are depictured, and in the filaments of the optic nerve which transmit these images to the brain? Hence it would allow; that as we receive different sensations of hot, cold, smooth, and rough, we should find the same difference in our sensations of colours, and the like.

In order for me to enter into your sentiments, said the Marchioness, you must explain what you mean by saying that the images of objects are depictured upon the membrane of the eye; and that the optic nerve transmits those images to the brain? Do you know, answered I, that an explication of this will be no less than an explication of a vision it self? So much the better, said she: indeed it seemed pretty strange to me, that after you had spoke so much upon the different ways in which it is possible for us to see, you should be silent upon the manner in which we really see. I will not defer this explication any longer, answered I, and I shall be extremely happy if my shewing you in what manner you see me, may induce you to look upon me in a different way from what you have hitherto done.

Light is principally subjected to the two accidents of *reflexion* and *refraction*. *Reflexion*, according to the Cartesians, happens when by collision of the globules of light with the solid parts of bodies, these globules are repelled back again, just as a ball rebounds when it is struck against the earth. And it is by this reflected light, that we see all bodies, the moon, the planets, heavens, and every thing else, except the sun, stars, fire, and all those other bodies here below, which shine by their own light. *Refraction* is caused when the globules of light in passing through air, water, glass, *etc.* meet with the pores and cavities of those bodies, so that the ray, which is only a chain or series of globules, breaks and is turned out of its proper path, and takes a different direction in its passage from what it had before. Pellucid or transparent bodies which suffer the light to pass through them, such as water, air, diamond, and glass, are called *mediums*. Hence *refraction* is said to happen when light passes from one *medium* to another. And this *refraction* is greater or less, that is, the rays are more or less broken and turned aside from their path, in proportion to the different densities of the *mediums* through which the light successively passes. Thus for example, the rays are more broken in passing from air into glass, than in passing from air to water, because glass is much more dense than water; and for the same reason they will be more broken in passing from air to diamond.

If this was a proper time, said the Marchioness, to make criticisms upon poets, it might be said, that Tasso has not expressed himself very accurately, when speaking of Armida, he says,

As limpid streams transmit the unbroken ray, etc.
Poetry, in these verses, does not seem to agree with optics, which will not allow that a ray can be transmitted unbroken. Tasso perhaps, answered I smiling, would be understood to speak of those rays which fall perpendicularly upon water or chrystal, that is, without being inclined, with regard to the surfaces of those *mediums*, either to one side or the other; as a threed would fall upon the ground if it had a weight fastened to it: for in this case the rays pass on without being broken, and continue to proceed in the same path as they first set out in: but the truth is, that poets do not address themselves to philosophers nor to you, who have nothing but *refractions* in your mind: but they write for the people, and consequently must often make use of vulgar prejudices and opinions. And provided the images be lively, the passions strong, and the num-

ers harmonious, we may pardon them a mistake in optics. What do you think of Ovid, who has perhaps stretched the poetic licence too far, and made the sun in a day run through all the signs of the Zodiac; whereas according to the exact rules of astronomy, his diurnal course is confined to about the thirtieth part of only one sign? In the second book of the *Æneis*, that master-piece of sublime poetry, there is a very fine image, which, if examined by the laws of optics, would lose all its justness. Æneas, after he had been assured by Hector in a dream of the irreparable ruin of his country, ascends a turret, and there discovers the treachery of the Greeks, whose dreadful effects appeared from every quarter. The palace of Deiphobus already levelled to the ground, his next neighbour Ucalegon on fire, and the flames of that city, which a ten years siege had attacked in vain, dreadfully reflected by the waves of the sea. Now in the situation in which Æneas stood this could not possibly be; for the opticians will tell you, that in order for him to see the flames of the city shine upon the sea, the sea must have been placed between him and those flames, which it was not. But who would not excuse this error, which can be seen only by a very few, for the sake of those fine verses which all the world admires?

But to return from poetry to physics, a transition which you have rendered very familiar to me, the manner in which the rays of light are broken in passing from a rare to a dense *medium*, as from air to glass, is different from what it is when they are transmitted from a dense to a rare *medium*, as from glass to air. I would be understood, always to speak of the rays which fall upon these *mediums* obliquely, and with some inclination; for as I mentioned to you before, those rays which fall perpendicularly do not suffer any deviation. If you suppose then, that a ray of light coming from the air should fall upon the surface of a glass, it will be broken in such a manner, that after its trajection, it will be less inclined to the surface of the glass, and immerging will approach nearer a perpendicular. After the same manner, a ray of light proceeding from your eye would strike the middle of this bason, provided it were dry. But supposing it filled with water as it now is, the ray could not continue its course directly to that point as at first, but in its transmission through the water would be bent in such a manner that it would fall on one side, and strike the bason in a point nearer to us. These are all the lines and figures that I will draw you, to explain the present subject.

What need is there of lines and figures, replied the Marchioness, to understand that a ray of light passing from air into water or glass, will be bent in going toward it, and approach nearer to a perpendicular? And does not the contrary happen, when the ray passes from glass into air? Yes certainly, answered I; the ray in this case is more inclined after its trajection to the surface of the air, which immediately touches the glass, it becomes more unlike a perpendicular, and places itself as it were behind the surface of the earth.

These *refractions* of the rays of light which were known though very imperfectly, to the antients, and to the consideration of which we in great measure owe the perfection of astronomy, are the cause of an infinite number of strange and amusing phænomena, which we every day observe such as objects appearing out of their place when viewed through a *prism*: an oar broken in the water, and the surprize of seeing ourselves deformed and crooked when in a bath.——This is the very thing, said she, interrupting ne, that I lately obferved when I was in the bath, and I was extremely furprized and puzzled to find out the reafon of it. It is nothing elfe, anfwered I, but the *refraction* which the rays fuffer in paffing from air into water. Thefe *refractions*, befides what we have already mentioned, are the caufe too why we fee the bottom of veffels and rivers much deeper than they really are, and that failors after a long and tedious voyage, have the pleafure of feeing and faluting the land, much fooner than they would otherwife do. This too is the reafon that the fun and full moon appear to our fight of an oval figure when near the horizon, and many other things of the like nature, which proceed from hence, that the rays in their paffage fiom thefe objects to our eyes are refracted, and come from places different from thofe where the objects themfelves are. The eye, which is not fenfible of thefe *refractions*, always refers and tranfports the objects to thofe places from whence the rays appear to proceed, or in other words, it fees them in the direction of the rays which penetrate and ftrike it. Hence it is, that the figure and fituation of things which are feen by refracted rays, come to be changed. If, without knowing any thing of the fcience of optics, the firft time I had the honour of feeing you, a *prifm* had been placed before my eyes, which by *refracting* the rays which proceed from you to me, had given them the fame direction which they would have had if they had come from the fky, you would certainly have appeared to me to have been tranfported into the world of chimeras, and incompaffed with an infinite variety of colours, and I fhould have intreated you to defcend, as Endymion did the moon, and addreffed myfelf to you in fome florid defcription of a fhady grove or lonely vale, in order to tempt you from the ftars. And all this fine delufion would have been occafioned by that direction which the *prism* had given to the rays, which would have flowed from you to my eyes.

I fancy, said the Marchioness, that mankind always look upon those, who are in a condition much superior to their own, through certain *prisms*, which make them appear as if they were transported to heaven, to revel upon ambrosia, enjoy the conversation of the gods, and be surrounded with glory and happiness; whereas the more they are elevated above others upon earth, the more subject are they to the sport and caprice of fortune. This comparison will appear still juster, answered I, upon this account, that as when we quit the *prism*, we see the objects again return to their proper place: so when we forsake the opinions of the vulgar, and substitute those of good sense in their room, these demigods appear nothing more than other men, and in a condition not greatly to be envied. But to return to our subject: A philosophical eye every day discovers an infinite number of strange and diverting phænomena arising from the change of direction produced in the rays of light, not only by *refractions* but by *reflexion* too. From hence proceed all the wonders of concave glasses, by the help of which, that poet, who wrote a dissertation on the nature of bees, could discern the small members and diminutive parts of that noble and industrious insect, and magnified them to that degree that each of *them seemed as big as a dragon*. With these glasses too the vestals rekindled their sacred fire, whenever it happened to be extinguished. From hence arose the fables of Archimedes and Proclus; and ignorance and imposture have rendered these glasses one of the favourite instruments of magic. But among the phænomena which arise from a change made by reflection in the rays of light, you will perhaps be furprized to find one which is every day prefent with you, and which perhaps you have never yet confidered as a phænomenon, much lefs a matter of wonder. What phænomenon can this be, faid the Marchionefs, to which I have paid fo little regard? It is, anfwered I, the image of your felf, which appears beyond the looking-glafs every morning, when you hold a confultation with the Graces in what manner it will be beft to give an artificial negligence to your hair. This reprefentation of your felf proceeds from hence, that all the rays, which flow from all the points of your face to the looking-glafs, are reflected in fuch a manner to your eye, as if they proceeded from as many other points as there are in your face, equidiftant from each other, and as far beyond the glafs, as you are of this fide of it; and confequently you fee your image at as great a diftance from the glafs, as you yourfelf are, and exactly like you; and from the pleafure this beauteous reprefentation affords you, you eafily conceive what pleafure the original muft give to others. The celebrated Milton has in his fublime poem finely defcribed the delight and furprize of Eve the firft time fhe furveyed herfelf in a fountain,

———*That flood unmov'd*
Pure as the expanfe of heav'n———.

And this image of herfelf appeared fo charming, that, like another Narciffus, fhe afterwards ingenuoufly confeffed to Adam, that though fhe thought him fair, yet he feemed,

——— ———*lefs fair*
Lefs winning foft, lefs amiable mild,
Than that fmooth wat'ry image———

Does not this paffage of Milton convey fome malicious insinuation, said the Marchioness? And is not his real meaning that the sight of a husband gives a woman less pleasure than even an image or a shadow? However, I agree that our first parent was in the right to admire this fine phænomenon, and I have been greatly to blame in my neglect of it; but we are too early accustomed to the sight of these things, for them to make a strong impression upon us. If any one had told me a few days ago, that certain rays, flowing from my face, would have been reflected from the looking-glass, I should have believed it to be one of those usual enigma's which gallantry borrows from tradition, or founded upon the authority of some old romance. But I confess that from this time, I shall survey myself in the glass with a sort of philosophical pleasure.

There is no greater pleasure, continued I, to philosophers, than that of observing the various sportings of the rays of light, in passing through a *gibbous* glass, or one that is convex on both sides, and from which its resemblance to a grain of *lentille*, is termed a *lens*. And upon this depends the explanation of vision. If two rays of light mutually *parallel*, that is to say, which always keep the same distance from each other without approaching nearer or removing farther off, like the espaliers of these walks, fall upon a *lens*, by means of that *refraction* which they suffer, they are united beyond it, into one point that is called the *focus of the lens*, which is more or less distant in proportion as the *lens* is more or less convex. So that the greater the convexity, the less will be the distance of the *focus*; and the less the convexity is, the distance of the *focus* will be the greater. And this distance of the *focus* is what distinguishes the *lens*: as for instance, we say this *lens* has so many feet of *focus*, and another so many, just is we say such a machine can raise the water to such a height, by which we would signify the force and activity of it. I fancy, said the Marchioness, that the reason why this point is called a *focus*, is because a candle may be set on fire when placed there, as I once saw done by a person who undertook to light a candle without the help of fire by the sun. He might safely have engaged, answered I, to light the candle not only without fire, but even with ice. For a *lens* made of ice in a little space of time produces the same effect as one that is formed of glass. How many impertinences might this have furnished the poets with in that time when their language was,

See guarded by the watchful powers of love,
Fair Delia *slumbers in the peaceful grove;*
Struck with the sight, let wond'ring mortals own,
Amidst the gloomy shades, a radiant sun!

But the reason that you give is a very good one: the burning which follows in that point where the *lens* unites the rays which were at first parallel, and forms them into a flame, is the very reason why it is called the *focus*. All the rays, which are not mutually parallel, but in going from a point keep continually removing from each other, and which are called *diverging* rays, unite beyond the *lens* in another point, which is always more distant than the *focus* of the *lens* itself. Hence we say, that a convex *lens* renders the parallel and diverging rays converging. For those rays are called *converging*, which proceeding from various parts, have a tendency to unite themselves in one point. Just as the alleys of those woods which are formed in the shape of stars, continually approach to one another till they all meet in the centre. These walks, said the Marchioness, interrupting me, might be called diverging, with

regard to one in the centre of the wood, from when[ce]
they proceed, always removing still farther from one an[o]-
ther. You only want, Madam, answered I, to turn ov[er]
Euclid and Apollonius a little, and sometime put on a[n]
abstracted look, and you will be a complete geometr[i]-
cian.

But to follow the tract of these rays as we have begu[n]
——the more that point, from which the diverging ray[s]
set out, is distant from the *lens*, the nearer the *lens* and i[ts]
focus is that point where the rays unite; and so on th[e]
contrary, the nearer that point from whence the divergin[g]
rays proceed is to the *lens*, the farther off from it and i[ts]
focus is that point where they unite; provided however
that the point from whence these rays proceed be not a[t]
such a distance, that instead of uniting they are thrown ou[t]
of the glass either diverging or parallel. Opticians, in order to find out the innumerable variations which these ray[s]
may form, make use of a certain science called *Algebra*
which after having extended its empire over all the region[s]
of natural philosophy, has since by the ingenious contriv[-]
ance of interest been appropriated to civil uses, to deter[-]
mine the chances of those games which are the most sub[-]
ject to the caprices of fortune, and has even insinuated it[-]
self into the litigious provinces of law and morality B[y]
the help of this science, they have always certain letter[s]
at hand, called symbols, connected with each other b[y]
certain signs: with these, provided they know the qualit[y]
of the *lens*, that is, the distance of its *focus* and of the poin[t]
from whence the rays proceed which fall upon the *lens*,
or the distance of the point to which the rays tend if they
should fall converging upon the *lens*, Opticians can tell
you in a moment, whether the rays will unite or not, whe-

On Light and Colours. 87

[eith]er they will go out of the *lens* diverging or parallel, and [at] what point they will unite. This looks like a species [of] magic, which perhaps would not have escaped unpunished in that age, when it was a crime to assert the motion [of] the earth, and the existence of the Antipodes.

The uniting of the rays diverging from several points, to the like number of points beyond the *lens*, which [se]ems in itself a very indifferent thing, supplies us with [on]e of the finest sights you can possibly imagine. If to [a] hole made in the window-shut of a darkened room, you [ap]ply a *lens*, and over-against this at a proper distance [th]ere be placed a sheet of white paper, you will see all the [o]bjects which are without the window, especially those [w]hich are directly opposite to the *lens*, inverted and painted upon the paper with a beauty, vivacity and softness of [c]olours that would make a landskip drawn by Claude Lorrain, or a visto by Canalleto, appear faint and languid. [Y]ou will perceive the distance of the objects exactly the [sa]me as you would do in a picture, that is, the smalness of [th]ose objects which are far off, from a little confusion and [o]bscurity, from a certain faintness of the colours, and in [sh]ort, from a most exact perspective the grand secret of [th]at happy art of delusion, painting, which accompanies [a]nd assists all I have been describing. It is impossible to [ex]press to you the pleasure that results from the motion [a]nd life which animates this fine piece: the trees are really [a]gitated by the wind, and their shadow follows the motion. [T]he flocks bound upon the lawns, the shepherd really [w]alks, and the sun-beams play upon the waters. Nature [d]raws her own picture inverted and in miniature.

It is pity, said the Marchioness, that so fine a picture [d]rawn by the hand of so excellent a master, should be turn-

H

ed upfide down, which I am as much at a lofs to find
reafon of, as I am of the manner in which it is form[ed].
Let us fuppofe, anfwered I, without fide of the wind[ow]
over-againft the *lens* an arrow to be placed horizontal[ly,]
that is, even with the bottom of the window: let the po[int]
of this arrow be on the right-hand, and the feathers on t[he]
left. Suppofe too that the extremity of the point em[its]
rays upon the *lens* which entirely cover it. Thefe ra[ys]
unite beyond the *lens* itfelf in another point, but in paffi[ng]
through the *lens*, inftead of being on the right hand
they were at firft, as proceeding from the point of the a[r]
row which we fuppofed to be on the right-hand, th[ey]
change their fituation, and are placed on the left. In t[he]
fame manner the extreme point of the feathers throws ra[ys]
upon the *lens* which unite in another point, and after the[ir]
paffage through the *lens* are turned from the left to t[he]
right hand. Juft in the fame manner as if a perfon hel[d]
two fticks, one in each hand, and fhould crofs them to[‐]
gether; that which before the croffing was on the rig[ht]
will afterwards be on the left-hand, and on the contra[ry]
that which was on the left will be on the right. No[w]
the rays, that fall upon the *lens*, crofs each other, juft a[s]
thefe two fticks do in the point where they touch. Th[e]
fame may be faid, if the arrow fhould be fet upright.
Thofe rays which proceed from the top of it, after bein[g]
croffed and paffing through the *lens*, remain at bottom
and thofe which came from the bottom at top. Thu[s]
you fee the whole fituation of the rays is changed. Tha[t]
which was at top is placed at bottom, and what was a[t]
bottom appears at top. That on the right-hand is turne[d]
to the left, and that on the left to the right. If a fhee[t]
of paper be then placed behind the *lens* in the place where

these rays unite, they will draw you an image of the arrow in which the point shall be on the left hand, and the feathers on the right, or in other words, the image will be the reverse of the object. You may easily transfer what I have said of the arrow, to a landskip, a piazza, or any other object, with this difference however, that all the parts of a landskip or piazza cannot be equally distinct in the picture as those of the arrow are, because the rays unite at different distances from the *lens*, in proportion to the different distance of the points from whence they flow. If, for instance, an object in the middle of this walk is seen distinctly upon the picture, as it will be if the paper be set in a place where the rays which come from it unite, those objects which are nearer cannot be distinct, because the point where the rays unite is at a greater distance; neither will those objects which are farther off be distinct, because the point where their rays unite is nearer the *lens*, and consequently the rays, as well of the one as the other, fall upon the paper disjoined, and only form an image there which will be very dim and languid, or in other words, confused; so that for those objects which are far off, we must place the paper nearer the *lens*, and set it at a greater distance when we should see those which are near.

It will now be necessary, said the Marchioness, that you should provide your self with a *lens*, and give me a sight of these fine landskips all round us upon a sheet of paper. For I must confess, I have a great curiosity for this, both as a woman, and as a woman whom you have rendered half a philosopher. I wish, answered I, that I had one with me to satisfy your curiosity this moment, which by what you say must be extremely strong. But I will satisfy you as soon as I am able with a view of this *camera obscura*.

H 2

But what will you imagine if I say to you when we are in it, suppose yourself to be placed in one of your eyes, and to see every thing that passes there?

The *camera obscura* represents the inside of our eye which is nearly of the shape of a ball: the hole in the window is the pupil which is in the fore-part of the eye and appears in all as a dark hole, sometimes greater, sometimes less. The *lens* is the chrystalline humour which is exactly of that figure, and is placed over-against the pupil, and suspended by certain little fibres called the ciliar processes, which proceeding from a coat or very thin skin which incompasses the inside of the eye, are fixed in the edge of it: the paper on which the image of objects is depictured, is the *retina*, composed of the filaments and medullary substance of the optic nerve, which is fastened to the eye behind, and is the great channel of communication between that and the brain. The spaces which are between the fore-part of the eye and the chrystalline humour, and between this and the *retina*, are filled with two humours less dense than the chrystalline, but denser than the air. By the help of all this *apparatus*, external objects are pictured upon the *retina* in miniature just as in the *camera obscura*, and thus we see.

Really I did not think, said the Marchioness, that I should be transported thus in an instant from the *camera obscura*, to the inside of my eye, nor that the fine picture, you before described, had so much relation to vision. Many must have observed this, answered I, before you, without suspecting any such relation. If there be a hole made in any room which is otherwise dark, and this hole does not exceed a certain bigness, this will be sufficient to shew you those objects which are over-against the hole, painted upon the oppofite wall or the floor of the chamber. Is there no need of the *lens* then, faith the Marchionefs, in order to the production of this picture? It is neceffary, anfwered I, to give it in fome meafure the finifhing ftroke. But even without the *lens* if the hole be fmall enough, and the oppofite wall or the floor not very diftant, the rays which pafs through the hole are near enough not to appear confufed, and may draw a tolerable picture of the external objects upon the wall or the floor.

If the chryftalline humour becomes opaque, which is that forms a cataract, there is no other remedy in this cafe to recover the fight, than by depreffing the chryftalline humour, and cutting away the fibres which hold it fufpended, and then fome faint reprefentation of the objects may be drawn on the *retina* of thofe unhappy perfons. But as the picture in the dark room is much weaker and more confufed if there be not a *lens* applied to the hole, fo is that which is made upon the *retina* of thefe perfons, when the chryftalline humour which is the *lens* of the eye is no longer fixed over-againft the pupil. It is true, thofe two humours which remain, the glaffy and aqueous, help the rays to unite, and a convex glafs may in fome meafure fupply the defect of the chryftalline humour. It would be well if this convex glafs could affift the eyes under a much more terrible diftemper, in which, though they feem well and found, the *retina* or the optic nerve being weakned and obftructed, cannot tranfmit any fenfation to the brain of the images of objects, though they are clearly and diftinctly drawn upon it. This diftemper, which is called a *gutta ferena*, occafioned the blindnefs, if not of the Greek, at leaft of the Britifh Homer, which he interweaves in his poem among the beauties of Paradise Lost, the battles of angels, and the pregnant abyss.

This picture then of the *camera obscura*, said the Marchioness, which seemed of no other use than to imploy idle people, or such as have a taste for painting, is in reality of very great service to us, and in some cases even restores sight to the blind. Are we not obliged to Des Cartes for having rendered it so useful to us? Des Cartes, answered I, is very happy, to whom you would willingly be obliged for every thing. But in this case your acknowlegements are due to an industrious German, who laid the foundation of many things which others have since brought to perfection. He was the first who gave us a true explication of Vision, which has always been a subject of speculation among philosophers; and consequently has had its share of ridiculous notions. For some among the ancients supposed certain rays, which, extending themselves from the inside of the eye to its superficies, pressed the air as far as the object to be seen; and this air finding some resistance from the object, made it perceptible to the sight; others affirmed that Vision was formed by the reflexion of the sight; that is, because rays flowed from the eye to the object, and were from thence reflected back to the eye; so that these gave it an exact information what the object was. Nor were there wanting some who affirmed that certain effluvia go from the eye, and meeting in their way with other effluvia of bodies, they link themselves with these, and turning back again with them to the eye, give the soul a perception of objects. And the most rational among them asserted, that extremely fine membranes formed of particles and atoms are thrown off from the surfaces of bodies, and have mutually the same disposition and order, as there is in the surfaces of the bodies themselves from whence they proceed, and that these membranes, which they call *simulachra*, or images exactly resembling the bodies from whence they are sent, enter into the eye, and this is the cause of our seeing. And it is surprising to think that in such an age as this, such a country as England, there should be found any person * who, shutting his eyes against the light of things, would be again immersed in the profound darkness of unintelligible words, and assert that Vision is formed by means of the different degrees of the expansive force communicated from bodies to the eye through a *plenum*, and that the different modifications of it, as clearness, weakness, and confusion in the sight, arise from the proportion which these expansive forces have with the contractile ones of the optic nerves. However, all the moderns except this, (who, like him that wrote in these latter ages against the circulation of the blood, was necessary to give us a specimen of the infinite varieties and extravagancies of the human mind,) have rejected these

---

* Dr. Robert Green, fellow of *Clare-hall*, Cambridge, published in 1712. a book intitled the *principles of natural philosophy*, in which is shewn *the insufficiency of the present systems to give us any just account of that science, and the necessity there is of some new principles in order to furnish us with a true and real knowlege of nature*. In this book he undertakes to shew the unreasonableness of the greatest part of that philosophy hitherto received under the name of the *Corpuscularian*, and then proceeds to lay down the principles upon which alone he thinks it possible for nature to be explained. He farther endeavours to evince the incompetency of the present mathematics to furnish us with any just or adequate reasonings upon nature, and the necessity there is of some new principles in that science, which he has in some manner explained in the *geometria solidorum* annexed to this book, and from which he has been long assured that the squaring of the circle is not impossible.———The celebrated Mr. Cotes professor of astronomy used to say that this book shewed the author to have had as extraordinary a genius as Sir Isaac Newton, since it must have been the effect of design to guard so effectually as he did against saying any one right thing throughout so large a treatise.

chimerical explications, the offspring of pride and ignorance; neither have they greatly esteemed the reasonings of those who thought that the effluvia proceeded rather from the eye, than from the objects; since it was more reasonable they should proceed from an animate than an inanimate substance; that the ears, the mouth, and the nose, were made concave to take these effluvia in, whereas the eye was made convex, and therefore proper to send them out. Notwithstanding all these fine reasons, opticians have reduced the eye to a perfect *camera obscura*, rejecting and extinguishing that light which the greater part of the ancients supposed to proceed from it. Indeed the august eyes of Tiberius must perhaps be excepted, who, as it is said, when he walked in the night, could for sometime see as well as in clear day light, which is said to arise from his emitting certain sparks from them. You may say the same thing of any other person, who is considerable enough to deserve that an exception should be made in his favour.

It will be necessary for us, said the Marchioness, to look upon cats as considerable persons, and make an exception in their favour too. We shall willingly grant them that honour, answered I, only they must not take it ill if we say that the light, which seems to proceed from their eyes in the dark, serves only to give light to objects, and by this means the image may be drawn upon their *retina:* for Vision, as well as innumerable other things, is performed in the same manner in men as in brutes; or rather we may acknowlege ourselves obliged to those for that evidence which we have of the manner of its operation: for in order to demonstrate it, we make use of the eye of an ox, or some other animal, at the bottom of which when the

LIGHT and COLOURS. 95

away, if we place a very thin and tran-
we shall see the image of those objects, to
is turned, drawn upon it and inverted, just
a *camera obscura*.

how very capricious our senses are. For
y that there is heat in the fire no less than

Thus we confound one motion which is
I another that it raises in our hands, with
f heat, which sensation is neither in the for-

. But we do not say that colour is in our
bjects, though without dispute the colours
ation and motion upon the *retina*, and are
t as strong and lively as they are upon the
ves. Thus we confound two things in the
ieat, and only one in that of colours.

said the Marchioness, that we are much
senses in this point, for exempting us from
least. But do not they amply repay them-
many others to which they have subjected
e see only one object, though it be looked
yes, and see it upright, though it be drawn
the eye. You are a little too much pre-
t the senses, answered I, and I must for
take their defence. Is not the reason of all
vhich you express against Vision, because
ie explanation of it from Des Cartes? De-
please, said she, without accusing me, and
I can, from the charge of these two illusions
against it. Would they not rather be illu-
I, if we were to see an object double which
single, and that to be inverted which we

know to be direct? To-morrow we will enter upon a discussion of these two points, which Huygens, one of the great promoters of knowlege in the last age, thought beyond the reach of human understanding. To-morrow perhaps you may know more than that great man, but it is impossible for *that* acquisition to render you more charming than you are to-day.

DIALOGUE III.

Several particulars relating to Vision, discoveries in Optics, and a confutation of the Cartesian *system.*

THE Marchioness felt the utmost impatience to be more learned than Huygens. She was not for losing a moment's time, but would have continued our discourses upon Vision, the next morning as soon as ever we were up. I told her that we must prepare ourselves with somewhat more ceremony for so high a degree of knowledge, and that it well deserved that we should at least wait till after dinner. In the interim not to lose time, she might learn how it comes to pass that the eye sees the objects which are without it, but cannot at all see itself. And from hence she might form a clearer idea of certain verses which no doubt must have been often addressed to her.

This was all the optics she could get from me in the morning. She waited for the afternoon with as much impatience, as an Initiate full of the expectation of being let into some profound mystery. In order to understand why we see only one object with two eyes, would you be pleased, Madam, said I, if I should tell you that in reality we see only with one eye, and that the other remains idle and at rest? You had better, said she, at once reduce us to a single eye, and then you will have no farther difficulty. I should be as well pleased, if you was to say that we walk only with one leg. You are more moderate, answered I,

than the Latin poet, who says, that women would b[e]
ill-pleased to have but one lover, as but one eye.
This strange explication however was given by a grave p[hi-]
losopher, and resembles the pride of the Chinese, w[ho]
fancy that all nations except their own see with but [one]
eye, since both the one and the other are equally the [off-]
spring of ignorance. But this may serve to let you [see]
what difficulties there are in solving the question we [are]
now upon. Another made the optic nerves to resem[ble]
two lutes composed of various strings, which have an [ex-]
act correspondence with each other, so that the two ima[ges]
of the object falling upon strings wound up to an equ[al]
height or a unison, the object must appear single. But [all]
these fine and ingenious explications will not make you [a]
better philosopher than Huygens. I believe that the tr[ue]
explanation of this difficult phænomenon, like many othe[rs]
in Vision, depends upon experiments. The senses of fee[l-]
ing and sight lend each other a mutual assistance in t[he]
formation of our ideas, just as our eyes and ears help eac[h]
other when we learn a new language. The sense of fee[l-]
ing, which is much stronger than the sight, has constantl[y]
informed us that in the ordinary way of seeing, the object i[s]
but one, and by a long habitude we join the idea of on[e]
single object with the two sensations of it. In the sam[e]
manner an object that is felt with two hands or two finger[s]
at a time, notwithstanding the two sensations which w[e]
have of it, seems to be only one; and this is occasione[d]
by those other ideas which we had conceived of it when w[e]
touched it only with one hand or one finger. If a butto[n]
or a ball of wax be pressed with two fingers at a time in a[n]
unusual manner, by crossing the fingers together, it wi[ll]
appear double, just as objects do when we squint upo[n]

[...]m. In both cases the antecedent ideas of feeling are [so] strongly united by a long habitude with these un[usu]al sensations, as to make us join them with the idea [of] one single object.

Do you believe then, said the Marchioness with an air [of] surprize, that if a person had been long accustomed to [pr]ess a button with two fingers crossed together, he would [no] longer feel it double? No certainly, answered I, for [th]e very same reason that objects do not appear double to [pe]rsons who are naturally squint-eyed. These by a long [u]se acquire the same habit in their manner of seeing as we [d]o in ours. We have a very singular and curious observa[ti]on to this purpose, upon a person who by some misfor[tu]ne had distorted and dislocated one of his eyes. At first [al]l objects appeared double to him, till at length by little [a]nd little, those which were the most familiar to him, that [i]s, those which he had the most experience of by feeling, [b]ecame single, and in time all the rest, though the dislo[c]ation still continued. I may venture to affirm that, by [v]irtue of this experience, Argus with all his hundred eyes did not see the fine heifer committed to his charge by the [j]ealous Juno, at all more multiplied than Polipheme did his Galatea with only one eye.

You seem to exult mightily, said the Marchioness, in this experience which we gain from our touch: will it give you confidence enough to undertake by its assistance the solution of that question I proposed to you yesterday: How it comes to pass, that objects, which are drawn inverted upon the eye, appear direct in the mind? These experiments, answered I, extend farther than you perhaps imagine, and the ideas of sight considered with regard to those which we received from touch, are no more than four

I

ftrokes of a pen compared to a fine *relief*. We have
example of a ftatuary, who though he was blind, yet
the help of his feeling made tolerable good likeneffes; o
of the greateft mathematicians in England, that land
phænomena, and who could give you a much better
planation of optics than I can, was yet deprived of
fight fo young, that he may be affirmed to have be
born blind. This perfon is certainly much more wonde
ful than that learned Frenchman, who, without eith
voice or ear, undertook to learn mufic, and very mu
improved the greateft and moft curious myfteries in th
art. Feeling furnifhes the imagination of this great ph
lofopher with much clearer and more diftinct ideas, tha
others receive from fight. What a pleafure would h
have in making ufe of your fine fingers to explain the con
verging and diverging of the rays? On the other hand
what could we learn, or what could we do without ou
feeling? We fhould be incapable to judge of the fituation
diftance, or figure of objects, as Berkley had prophefied
who perhaps confidered the metaphyfics of Vifion more
than any one ever did; and experience has verified this in
fome perfons, who, after being cured of cataracts born
with them, could not form any judgment, till the touch
lent them its affiftance; without this, our eyes would continually tantalize us with a view of knowlege and pleafure,
which we could never enjoy. The daily experiments then,
that we make with our feeling, inform us that objects are
direct, in the fame manner as they teach us they are fingle,
that they are placed in certain fituations, at certain diftances, and of certain figures. I believe Des Cartes is the
only one who ever pretended to give an immediate explication of this difficult phænomenon by a fimilitude. Sup-

d he, to have two sticks across each other,
t, and the other in the left hand, and to
eyes shut about a room with these sticks
ere is no question but you will think those
touch with the stick in your right-hand,
is means will make a pressure upon that
le left; and in like manner whatever you
ther stick in the left-hand, you will affirm
it. After the same manner the rays which
jects to the bottom of the eye, crossing
e chrystalline humour, those which press
right side will make you refer those points
y proceed to the left side, and those rays
n the left you will refer to the right side;
ays, which press upon the upper parts of
make you refer the points from whence
the lower part, and those of the lower to
d by this means the image, which is in
retina, makes you see the objects direct.
he Marchioness, this is very ingenious;
confine ourselves to this without seeking
it gives us an immediate explication of
a? Experience, answered I, unhappily
t this is not an ingenious explication: a
upon his head sees every thing inverted,
the images of external objects are pictured
in the very same manner when he is in
they are when he stands upon his feet.
idea of high and low, than what regards
; and when he is in this inverted positithe whole universe to be so too. Besides,
of Des Cartes supposes the idea of high

and low, right and left, which we can only have fro[m]
feeling, to be antecedent.

It is our feeling, which by an experiment every mom[ent]
repeated has constantly taught us to call the earth, t[o]
wards which we find ourselves continually carried by g[ra]
vity, *low*, those things which are contiguous to the eart[h]
as the pedestal of a pillar or our feet, *below;* and th[e]
things which are distant from the earth, *above;* as o[ur]
head or the top of a tree. The sense of feeling conve[ys]
these and the like ideas into the soul of a man born blin[d]
with as much exactness as that of sight does the ideas [of]
colour into ours. Now, if we suppose that vail whi[ch]
hides the visible world from his sight, to be taken aw[ay]
all at once, and consider in what manner he would jud[ge]
of the situations of objects, we might from thence arrive [at]
a clear knowlege of the manner in which we ourselves jud[ge]
of them, since we have the ideas of high and low in co[m]
mon with him: he would certainly be more surprised [at]
first opening his eyes, than the famous * Epimenides w[ho]
after his long sleep of so many years, who remember[ed]
nothing which he saw about him when he walked, n[or]
even the place where he had been born and brought u[p]
A new scene of ideas displays itself to him, a torrent [of]
new perceptions rush upon him through this new aven[ue]
by which objects enter the soul. Amazed and overwhel[med]

* A Cretan philosopher, when he was a boy, being sent by [his]
father into the country, to fetch a sheep, he turned out of the ro[ad]
at noon, and reposed himself in a cave, where he slept 57 years. [Af]
ter this refreshment he awaked and looked about for the sheep, im[a]
gining he had slept but a little while; not finding it, he procee[ded]
to his father's country estate, where he saw every thing altered a[nd]
in possession of another He then returned to the city, and w[ent]
to his father's house, where his younger brother, now grown an [old]
man, at last knew him, and gave him an account of all that h[ad]
happened. He was held in great veneration among the Gree[ks]
who imagined him a peculiar favourite of heaven. He is said to h[ave]
lived till 150 years old, or, according to others, 297.

d with them, he finds himself transported, without knowing how, into another world. What a pleasure, what an extasy must this be, said the Marchioness! If novelty which always hovers about these things of which we have an idea, and is nothing more than an unusual combination of those objects we are already acquainted with, affords so much delight, what an infinitely greater pleasure must this man have in a world of things really new, and a new combinations of those ideas which he before had joined to those, with which the addition of another sense abundantly supplies him. But as human happiness is too often attended with some alloy, is it not possible for him to see something that would make him wish his eyes shut again when they were hardly open? He would have great reason to believe, that those objects would appear pleasing to this new sense, which had been so to the rest, and flatter this as agreeably as they had done those. But might not the event happen quite contrary to his expectation? And those objects, which had delighted his touch and hearing, prove very disagreeable to his sight? So that instead of increasing the number of his pleasures, this new sense would deprive him of the most sensible of them, and perhaps cruelly dissolve some pleasing tye which the others had closely bound.

It is true, answered I, that these senses do not always agree: how many persons do we daily see, who, convinced by sorrowful experience, that the reality of things does not agree with their outward appearance, find themselves too soon in possession of what they once thought they could never obtain soon enough? A blind man, answered the Marchioness, at least, while he is in love, should never desire to see; satisfied in the judgment of those senses which

reprefent an object agreeable to him, why fhould he
that of another, which perhaps would at once cond[e]
his choice, and, like reafon, probably make him fee
misfortune without giving him any affiftance to avoid
The only confolation, anfwered I, that this miferable p[er]
fon could have under the misfortune of fight is, that
would not be unhappy fo foon as you perhaps imag[ine]
How! faid fhe, if the joy of receiving his fight did
entirely deprive him of all complaifance, would not
very firft thing he defired to fee be that perfon for wh[ose]
fake he principally wifhed for the fight of his eyes? A[nd]
when he had feen her, he would immediately, if fhe fho[uld]
appear difagreeable, perceive his unhappinefs, if with
gard to beauty, love did not render him a fecond ti[me]
blind. He would enquire for her, anfwered I, would
her, and yet would not by that means know her aga[in].
This would be a miracle even beyond the power of love
effect; he would hear, if you will, the found of thofe wor[ds]
pleafing to his ear, and ftill more pleafing to his hea[rt]
but he would not know the mouth from whence they pr[o]
ceeded. Yet more, he would be fo far from diftinguifhi[ng]
another, that he would not diftinguifh himfelf, his ow[n]
feet or hands, from any affiftance his new fight cou[ld]
give him, fince he muft be utterly ignorant of the co[n]
nexions which the perceptions of fight have with thofe [of]
the touch; yet this connexion is abfolutely neceffary in ord[er]
for his knowing thofe objects again of which he had no ide[a]
but what he received from fenfes of a nature very differe[nt]
from that of fight, and depends upon an experiment whic[h]
he has never yet made. His own hands would be the fi[rst]
object he would learn to diftinguifh, by touching and loo[king]
ing upon them at the fame time, and remembering th[at]

such an idea of his feeling would agree with such another of his sight. When he had learnt this short lesson, love would the more easily conduct him to those experiments that would soon, either to his joy or sorrow, satisfy his curiosity, and we will conduct him to those that may content us, which is of a more philosophical nature.

One of the first he would try, would be to lift up that hand which he has now no trouble to distinguish, and in doing this, he would perceive some change in the situation which he received of it from his sight, and the reason of this change is because the image changes its situation in the *retina*, in proportion as the hand is higher or lower. Guided by nature herself, he would diligently observe what sort of sensation he felt when he held his hand up, and whenever he felt the same sensation raised in him, either by the same or any other objects whose image would fall in the same situation of the *retina*, though unknown to him, he would conclude that object to be high, or in that situation in which his hand at first was. By this means connecting the old ideas of feeling, with the new ones of sight, he judges of the height or lowness of the object, of its being direct or inverted; and it is of no importance, whether the image of this object be pictured upon the *retina*, direct, or inverted, or in any other position.

External objects are *signified* to him, if I may use that expression, by certain sensations of light and colours, as the thoughts of the soul are to us by certain characters, not by virtue of any resemblance between the one and the other, but by means of an arbitrary, yet constant and perpetual, connexion which we have observed between them. And as when we are accustomed to any particular manner of writing, it makes no change in the order of the ideas which these characters excite in us, whether they be written from left to right, as ours are, from right to left like the Oriental, or from top to bottom after the Chinese manner; so whether certain images be drawn direct or inverted upon the *retina*, it does not at all change our judgment of their situation.

The blind person, who has hitherto safely conducted us through this labyrinth, resembles each of us. We enter into light with our eyes shut, and probably do not begin to *see* till we have for sometime *felt*. Thus, Madam, you are indebted to the predominant sense of feeling for this new explication too, and however little you may imagine it, you will find that to this you have had the greatest obligations through the whole course of your life.

I see very plainly, said she, that you interest yourself for the honour of the touch, much more than for that of Des Cartes; and it is not possible to propose any difficulty but you will be ready to give it a solution by the help of this sense. There are other difficulties, answered I, which I will give you a solution of without this, that you may see I have great plenty of explications. One of these perhaps may be to know what change must be made in the eye, in order for it to have a distinct view of objects placed at different distances. For as in the *camera obscura*, the rays which flow from objects that are near unite at a greater distance from the *lens*, than the rays of those which are more remote; so the very same thing happens in the eye, where the rays, which proceed from the pillars of this gallery, unite at a greater distance from the chrystaline humour, than those that come from these trees which are farther from it: what change then must be made in the eye, in order that when we look upon thefe trees, after having looked upon the pillars, the rays which proceed from them may be united upon the *retina*, or in other words, that we may have a diftinct view of them? The *retina*, anfwered fhe, muft be brought nearer the chryftalline humour, juft as the paper in the *camera obfcura* is brought nearer the *lens*, in order to give us a diftinct image of the more remote objects.

You have hit upon the true explanation, anfwered I; and fome have affirmed, that certain mufcles, which incompafs the eye, are made ufe of to produce this effect, and prefs the *retina* farther back from the chryftalline humour, or bring it more forward, as different occafions require. Thefe mufcles have befides another office, and help us to lift up or deprefs the eye, to turn it to the right or left, and give it a certain oblique motion which Venus has the principal care of regulating. Others have fuppofed that the *retina* remains immoveable, and that the chryftalline humour approaches nearer to it, and removes farther off, or that the chryftaline humour only changes its figure, growing more convex for near objects, and lefs fo, for thofe which are diftant; and others have affirmed, that each of thefe happens at the fame time, which will produce the fame effect, as if the *retina* approached to or receded from the chryftaline humour; but you had better fuppofe this latter, becaufe it is eafieft to imagine. For every diftance then, there is required a new conformation in the eye, and becaufe this cannot be effected without motion, and a certain effort, fome are of opinion that the eye informs us of the various diftances of objects by a certain natural geometry. But this way of judging, efpecially where very diftant objects are concerned, is extremely uncertain, as indeed almost all the rest are which have ever appeared upon the stage of philosophy.

But however this be, there are some persons who cannot bring their *retina* so near to the chrystaline humour as is necessary, in order to give them a distinct view of distant objects. There are others, who, on the contrary, cannot press it back far enough, to make objects which are near appear distinct. The first of these, who are vulgarly called short-sighted, are by opticians named *myopes*, and the second, commonly called long-sighted, *presbytæ*: these may be considered as the extremes betwixt which that sight, which is called just and perfect, stands. Notwithstanding the honour of being distinguished by names drawn from Greek, these persons could not help perceiving they had a defect in their eyes, which led them to seek for some remedy: the *myopes* in order to have a distinct view of distant objects, and the *presbytæ* of those at hand. These last found relief in convex-glasses, which, applied to the eyes, removed their defect; for these making those rays to become converging, which would without their assistance have fallen diverging upon the chrystalline humour, unite them at a less distance than they would otherwise have done; and the image of those objects which are opposite to the *lens*, is drawn distinctly upon the *retina*. The *myopes* found their remedy in concave glasses which disperse the rays and make them diverge; contrary to the convex ones, which make the diverging rays become converging. These concave-glasses then give a disposition to the rays, as if they came from a nearer object than they really do, and applied to the eye of a *myope*, they in a certain manner transport the distant object to a nearer situation, and thus a distinct image of it is drawn upon his *re-*

ina; for there is nothing more required to give short-sighted persons a distinct view of any thing, than to bring [it] nearer to their eye.

It was very happy for them, replied she, to find these glasses as safe and easy a remedy perhaps as ever the art of physic itself invented. But what did they do before they were found out? Till the thirteenth century, answered I, when these glasses are supposed to be invented, the Myopes were obliged to approach near to distant objects in order to see them distinctly, hoping perhaps that an advanced age, when according to the common opinion the *retina* approaches nearer to the chrystalline humour, might give them some relief from this inconvenience; but indeed this is a remedy much worse than the disease. The Presbytæ, on the other hand, were obliged to remove a great way off, without any hope of ever seeing the objects situated near them distinctly, if they should at any time have a curiosity for it, and they continually tormented their eyes with plaisters and *collyria*, without gaining the least advantage to their sight. I think the condition of these last, said the Marchioness, much more to be pitied than that of the first, both because they cannot flatter themselves with the least hope of growing better, and because they lose a great deal more in the conversation of ladies than the Myopes do. How miserable must have been the state of a poor Presbyta, who could never have a distinct view of his mistress, unless he breathed his sighs ten foot distant from her!

These are not so much to be pitied, answered I, as you imagine, since this defect generally happens in an age when hope and the conversation of ladies naturally desert us. For this is a defect of old men, as the very word Presbyta imports. But there are other defects and infirmities of t[he] sight incident to all ages, which are never placed in th[e] number of defects, for the very same reason that the fol[ly] of being more solicitous for the future than the presen[t,] and by that means continually procrastinating our happ[i]ness, is never reckoned among the list of follies, namel[y,] because it is common and universal. Philosophers, wh[o] have a quicker perception of things, have discovered a[nd] sought remedies for these defects; one of which is, th[at] very small objects are invisible, however near they may [be] placed to the eye; the other, that very distant objects ca[n]not be discerned, even if they are of a very great magn[i]tude. These are inconveniences which you see are not [at] all felt by the vulgar, but reserved for the curiosity a[nd] nice perception of philosophers. The reason of both d[e]fects is, because the image of very small or very distant o[b]jects, painted upon the *retina*, is not big enough to [be] perceived by the eye, notwithstanding the proximity of t[he] one, or extraordinary magnitude of the other. The r[e]medies invented by philosophers to supply them are certa[in] instruments, whose only business is to magnify this ima[ge,] and render it perceptible to the eye, by means of vario[us] combinations of glasses, or by one alone. Those whi[ch] are made use of to discern distant objects, are called *tele*copes, and those which help us to a sight of exceeding sm[all] objects, *microscopes*. We are obliged to each of these f[or] an infinite number of discoveries, which could never ha[ve] been made without them. The heavens are the princip[al] object of the *telescope*, from whence it has furnished philoso[*]phers with more curiosities than ever Columbus could brin[g] from America to enrich the cabinets of the naturalist[s.] For not to speak of the hills and vallies which they ha[ve]

in the moon, the fatellities of Jupiter fo very
:ography, thofe of Saturn with his *ring*, it is to
opes that we owe our difcovery of the fpots in the
er, and Mars, which are neceffary in order to
the periods of their revolution round themfelves,
: affiftance of thefe, aftronomers have given us
nap of Venus, that they are as well acquainted
mountains in heaven, as the geographers are
upon earth. They have difcovered that this
an increafe and decreafe, that it is at one time
.nother full, in fhort, that its appearance and
ictly refemble thofe of the moon, as it had been
d by the celebrated Copernicus, before the in-
the telefcope. Thefe give the celeftial bodies
)er diftances, and have fhewn us an infinite num-
rs, unknown to the antients, difcovering fo great
r in the milky-way, as is fufficient to fupply ten
worlds befides our own. In fhort they have
a true fyftem of our world, by extending its confinity; fo that if a poet, to flatter a nation which
: a greater progrefs in the conqueft of the world,
he knowlege of its frame, could fay, that when
irned his eyes upon our earth, he could fee no-
it that was not fubject to the Roman empire, we
n with greater truth, that if he looked upon the
or at leaft the *folar vortex*, he could not fee any
it, but what is the difcovery and conqueft of the

prefent thefe telefcopes to me, replied the Mar-
under fuch fublime images, that I am afraid the
)es will make but a very infignificant figure, when
l to them. There is, anfwered I, **a** very remark-

K

able difference between them, in which I believe the[y] have the advantage. The telescopes, it is true, by [dis]covering to us the hills and valleys in the planets, their [mo]tions, revolutions round their own axis, that is to say, th[eir] day and night, the moons that from time to time sup[ply] the absence of the sun; in short, by representing them [to] be of the same nature as our earth, have furnished us w[ith] materials to people these vast and immense bodies wh[ich] were before uninhabited, stood neglected in a corner [of] the universe, and were believed to exist for no other [end] than to please our eyes. But microscopes have made us [in] reality see an infinite number of animals, of which we h[ad] not the least knowlege before, in things which were [not] looked upon as very proper to afford them a habitati[on.] Not to say any thing of the discoveries in anatomy and n[a]tural history, which we owe to these glasses; aromatic [in]fusions, a drop of vinegar, are peopled by so prodigio[us] a number of little animals, that Switzerland and Chi[na] would appear empty and uninhabited, when compared [to] them. The microscope, said she, is the compass of ph[i]losophy; each of these have given their assistance to t[he] discovery of new worlds; the only difference is, that t[he] microscope has lent its art to people, and the compass [to] destroy.

It is very wonderful, answered I, into what innumerab[le] animal worlds philosophers have penetrated, under t[he] guidance of this compass. It is an amazing thing to r[e]flect upon the minuteness, art, and curiosity of the joint[s,] bones, muscles, tendons, and nerves necessary to perfor[m] the swift motions of the smallest microscopical animals.

These discoveries shew us in how little a compass all a[rt] and curiosity may be comprized, even in a body less th[an] small grain of sand, and yet as complete, as exquisitely formed, and as finely adorned, as that of the largest animal. Their multiplicity is no less surprising than their extreme smalness. A drop of the green scum upon water, no bigger than a pin's head, will contain no fewer than a hundred; which, far from being confined in that narrow extent, play about in it with all the freedom imaginable. The eye of a butter-fly will contain more than twenty-four millions of eyes; and the wonder is still greater, when we come to consider the organization of their fine and minute parts. If the eye of a fly, which seems to be a little misformed protuberance, be looked on thro' a microscope, it appears to be only a composition of thousands of little eyes, just as some nubilous stars, on being viewed with a telescope, appear to be a cluster of innumerable other stars. In some insects there have been counted no less than thirty four thousand of these little eyes, which, notwithstanding their extreme smalness, had each of them a chrystalline humour as perfect as ours.

Why are not our eyes, said the Marchioness, of so fine a texture? This question, said I, has been already answered.

For this plain reason, man is not a fly.
Say to what use were finer optics given?
To inspect a mite, not comprehend the heav'n.

But in fact, there are some insects, that with these microscopic eyes can see as far as the greatest part of men. The bees, an industrious species of flies, from whose labour we reap so great an advantage, can direct themselves safely to their hives, though at a mile distance, when they return laden with the sweet treasures of the spring. It appears that what nature has given us in reason, she has de-

nied us in exquisiteness of sense. Pigeons, the cour[iers]
of the east, such as that which brought news from Eg[ypt]
to Jerusalem, when it was besieged, of a quick and pow[er]
ful succour, or that beautiful one presented by Venus [to]
Anacreon in exchange for one of his odes, and whi[ch]
for having so often carried his letters to Bathyllus, deser[ved]
to sleep, and be sung upon that lyre which could resou[nd]
nothing but love; these flying couriers, I say, being l[et]
loose by the person, who has a mind to send home ne[ws]
of himself, ascend a prodigious height, and from thenc[e]
though at a very great distance, can see their native cou[n]
try, and safely direct their flight to it, without the he[lp]
of either stars or compass. Moles seem to be quite co[n]
trary to these sharp-sighted couriers. Nature, said t[he]
Marchioness, has perhaps made them amends some oth[er]
way. It is probable, that she has constituted the cond[i]
tion of animals pretty near as equal as that of men. The[ir]
eyes, answered I, are certainly not to be envied: they a[re]
so small, and covered with hair, that it seems as if natu[re]
had given these tenants of darkness, eyes to see the ligh[t]
for no other end than to fly from it. These animals ar[e]
not formed to contemplate the wonders of the microscop[e]
nor see in one drop of water so many thousands of animals
organized with that exactness which is necessary to enabl[e]
them to see, move, and nourish both themselves and othe[r]
little animals, which repay them the mischief they do t[o]
us, and to contain within them an infinite number of sti[ll]
other little animals of their own species, much less than
they, and which only wait to unfold themselves to make
their appearance in the microscope. These observations
open a scene of innumerable other worlds of animals unknown before, which, notwithstanding their extreme and

surprizing smalness, have their greater and less, their elephants and ants, just as ours has; the only difference is, that our ants become elephants when compared with their largest animals, or rather are as the immense distance of Saturn from us, is to the extent of a grain of sand.

Indeed, said the Marchioness, this new scene of pigmy worlds gives me as much pleasure, as that other immense and gigantic scene of *vortices*, or suns diffused over the whole universe. The little has its beauties as well as the great, or rather, answered I, there is no great or little, but with regard to ourselves. Gulliver, who could destroy the Liliputians like so many flies, was among the Brobdinagians kept in a cage like a Canary bird, or for an ornament upon the chimney, like a Chinese pagod. It is principally the microscope, and that infinite number of pigmy worlds discovered by it, which has rectified our ideas of great and little so much, that I am persuaded, that the consideration of this incredible and surprising smallness, which it has rendered perceptible to our senses, has served to soften and familiarize to mankind another consideration which is the master-piece of human understanding, and directly leads us to the subversion of great and small. This is the consideration of infinitely small quantities, which has made so great a noise in the learned world, and which you perhaps may have heard of. The meaning of this expression is, that there are parts and quantities in extension, so exceedingly small, that they may be reckoned as nothing when compared with our measures, as the fathom, foot, inch, and the like. So that if one of these quantities was added to the extremity of a line, for example, of a foot, it would not increase the length of it, nor decrease it if it was to be taken away. And the

K 3

mathematicians affirm, that in these quantities, infinitely small with regard to the ordinary measures called *differences*, there are innumerable orders and gradations, that a quantity, which is infinitely small compared with the order of our common measures, is infinitely great when compared with an inferior order of infinitely small quantities, and so of the rest. The most enormous size we have may become infinitely small when compared with an order of greatness infinitely superior. To how small a size is reduced the colossus of Nero, or that of Rhodes when compared to mount Athos, carved in the shape of man, and holding a city in one hand, and pouring out a river in the other? Compared to Milton's Satan, Virgil's Fame, the formidable Shade of * Camoens, that Polephem of the ocean, which appeared to the Portuguese sailors, his its head in the clouds, and its feet in the unfathomable abyss of the sea; or in short, what would all this appear to that angel seen by Mahomet in his mysterious night, whose eyes were seventy thousand days journey distant from each other? It is computed that if he were of a human shape there must be the distance of forty thousand years journey from his head to his feet.

Probably, said the Marchioness, there must be a great number of telescopes and speaking-trumpets in the Turkish paradise, in order for the Mahometans to be able to see and converse with these diabolically great angels of theirs,

* Camoens, the famous Portuguese poet, in his Lusiada, the subject of which is the discovery of the East Indies by his countrymen, conducts their fleet round the coast of Africa, and as it sails in sight of the Cape of Good Hope, he introduces a formidable spectre walking in the depth of the sea, its head reaching to the clouds, its arms extended over the waves, and its whole form surrounded with clouds, storms, winds, thunders, and lightenings. This spectre is the guardian of that foreign ocean which no ship had ever passed through before, complains of his being obliged to submit to fate, and the bold undertakings of the Portuguese, and foretels them the misfortunes they must undergo in the Indies.

There are, answered I, the same orders of infinites in the succession of time, as there are in extension. An hour, a minute, a second, are of an infinite duration compared with periods of time infinitely shorter. How enormous must the duration of the Roman empire seem to an animal, which in the space of five or six hours is born, grows up, produces one like itself, becomes old, and dies? What we should call the flight of time, would seem to this insect an eternity. But what are these durations of empires, this long succession of kings, emperors, consuls, and these tedious sieges, when compared with eternity? Is it more than a point in which we live, fight, raise such great commotions, and make so much noise? The Orientals say, there is a god that governs this world, who dies at the end of a hundred thousand years, and this space another superior God esteems but as a minute. And yet all these examples give us but a very imperfect idea of infinity. This consideration, the utmost stretch of the human mind, which we owe to Sir Isaac Newton, and which entirely overthrows all the ideas of absolutely great or little, was the foundation of the famous arithmetic of *fluxions*, or infinitely small quantities, which transplanted geometry into a province entirely new. Here it made so rapid and great a progress, that all it had done before seems nothing, and here by the assistance of new discoveries it produced such strange paradoxes, that they have in some measure clothed truth in the agreeably surprizing dress of fiction: and what is the most remarkable in the new geometry is, that by considering the properties, relations, and habitudes between infinitely small quantities, it arrives at the discovery of common and finite measures, which are the object of our enquiries.

If the sagacity which we so much admire, said she, consists principally in uniting those things in the mind, and finding their relation, which seem to be in their own nature disjoined and separated, what an unlimited understanding must Sir Isaac Newton have had to find the relation, and in some measure unite these quantities, disjoined and separated from each other by the immense tracts of infinity, where the human imagination quite loses itself! And, continued I, the consideration of these infinitely small quantities that we neither see, nor can conceive, which appeared only fit to perplex geometry, have in fact served to render it more easy, and reduced it at the same time to such general rules, that the most sublime and abstruse truths, in this science, are at present nothing but one of the infinite consequences which is lost among the croud of those that are deduced from the stroke of a pen; and, if you please, in a circle of ladies; truths that once required an Archimedes, with all that attention of thought which was necessary to make a person insensible of the noise of a town taken by storm, and be knocked on the head without perceiving it.

This consideration then of infinitely small quantities, said the Marchioness, and the observations of the microscope, which have rendered it more familiar and common, have given a very strange turn to geometry. It now treats of quantities, which from their extreme smalness were once utterly unknown, and does not at present disdain to enter into the company of ladies. A province with which I believe it was once as little acquainted, as with that of the infinitely small quantities. It is true, answered I, that geometry is rendered so very familiar, as sometimes to suffer itself to be treated by a hand as beauteous as that of

Venus of Medicis. But it is true likewise, that it sometimes resumes its fierce and savage disposition, especially when it is attended by that train of consequences, deduced from the stroke of a pen, as I before mentioned to you, and goes back into solitude and retirement.

Mankind however, said she, ought to think themselves greatly obliged to the microscope, for having contributed to soften and familiarize a thing whose very name alone inspired so much terror. Mankind, answered I, are not very often guilty of the sin of gratitude, and, as that polite philosopher, who is to instruct you in the motion of the earth, observes, there are some who make no scruple to treat the study of anatomy, which perhaps may have saved their lives, as a useless thing. You may judge from hence, whether it be probable that mankind will be grateful at the expense of so much consideration as is necessary in order to know whether the microscopes have contributed any thing to familiarize the calculation of infinitely small quantities, what this calculation is, and what uses it may have; all which things are necessary to form a well-grounded and rational gratitude. An English frier, called Roger Bacon, who lived in the thirteenth century, and had a general knowlege of the effect of the *refractions* of light by a *lens*, and was besides acquainted with many other things which are commonly believed to be the production of much latter ages, such as the invention of gun-powder, the reformation necessary to the calendar, and was sensible of the false method of study at that time in fashion; this very man, worthy of a statue and immortal honours, was ill treated, persecuted, kept prisoner for many years, accused as a conjurer and wizard, and of holding intelligence with the Devil, in order to effect what required only superior parts, and a free use of reason; and all the honour, these inventions, which we at present so greatly admire, met with at that time was, that the inventor was judged worthy to be burnt alive. It is true, that at present the learned cannot admire the depth of understanding, and the quick penetration of a man, who, in so barbarous an age as the thirteenth century, thought in a manner that very few of his species do even in this age, as enlightened as it is. But what gratitude is this to persecute, imprison, and almost burn him when living, and at the end of five centuries, to republish and give him the highest encomiums? Is not this like deifying Homer after his death, when he had been suffered to starve with hunger, while living? The telescopes, which have been the cause of so many fine discoveries in the heavens by their assistance, did not by that means at all advance his fortune here upon earth.

It is surprising, said the Marchioness, to see the folly and caprice of mankind. In some cases they are so extremely fond of novelty, as to adopt the most extravagant things merely on that account. This, we see, happens, every day in the fashion of dress, fitting, taking snuff, and even sneezing. At another time, novelty is an objection to the most useful and well contrived schemes. Are our judgments never to be guided by reason?

The wise men of past ages, answered I, appear to us like the moon just on the edge of the horizon, and those of the present time, like the same planet, when it is a great way above it. The image of the moon painted on our *retina*, when she is at the horizon, is less than when she is elevated a great way above it, at the meridian, for example; and this is occasioned by the distance of the moon from us, which is greater in the first case than the second.

On LIGHT and COLOURS.

Yee notwithstanding this, we imagine her to be much bigger at the horizon than at the meridian. This mistake proceeds from the interposition of other objects, as trees, houses, tracts of land, sea and sky, which are betwixt us and the moon, when at the horizon, but not when she is at the meridian, for in that situation she is left entirely to herself. Now as the objects placed betwixt us and the moon, make us imagine that she is more distant from us at the horizon, than the meridian, they are the reasons too why we imagine her to be bigger, because the apparent bigness of an object depends on the size of its image on the *retina*, joined to the judgment we form of its distance; so that the image being always of the same size, the object must appear so much the greater, as it is judged to be more distant. Hence it is, that actors, when they come from the bottom of the theatre, appear to us like giants, the perspective and the delusion of the scene making them appear a great way off. Why should those objects placed betwixt us, and the moon when at the horizon, said the Marchioness, interrupting me, make us imagine her to be farther off from us, than when she is at the meridian? I should think they would rather make her seem nearer, for in that situation she appears to touch them, and it seems probable she should appear at the same distance from us as the objects themselves; whereas at a greater altitude, we see her placed in the sky, and consequently judge her to be at a great distance. We know, answered I, that the moon in both cases is in the heavens, or rather that the heavens themselves are an immense vault, to which our imagination always refers the heavenly bodies. But the sky itself seems much more distant from us at the horizon, than when we look directly above our heads, so that it appears to us as a compressed vault. Between us and the part of the heavens which is over our heads, there is nothing to regulate our judgment of its distance; whereas at the horizon the long series of intermediate objects help us to form the distance, and make us judge it very great. Hence it comes to pass, that distances appear much greater upon a plain than a mountain; because the equality of the plain lets us see every thing that is placed between us and the distant object, which the inequality of the mountain will not suffer us to do.

In the famous picture of Correggio, at Parma, so ill copied by the chizel of Agostius Caracci, who was otherwise a great man in his profession, an artful series of hands, heads and feet, place a distance between St. Catharine and the head of the Madona, so sensible, that you would imagine it might be measured by the touch, and which, added to the other beauties and graces of art all united there, render it a master-piece of painting.

Now, to finish our optic comparison, the antients appear to us through a long series of emperors, kings, archons, consuls, and many other objects, which greatly magnify them: but we see the moderns alone, separated and left entirely to themselves like the moon at the meridian. Hence it is, that the manner in which the antients buttoned their coats, will be a subject of admiration to the learned, whereas there will be only two or three men of good sense to applaud any useful invention of a modern, who has the misfortune to be born in the same age with ourselves, and not to be distinguished by a name with a Greek termination. And this is the way in which a great part of those who value themselves upon their learning, think. Horace very finely satirized this folly in the time of Auguus. So true is it, that a wrong turn of thinking is the growth of every age.

But would not the Chinese, said the Marchioness, be gainers by the immense distance between them and us? And may not a million of miles produce the same effect as many successions of kings and consuls? They are certainly no losers by it, answered I: but however, those very persons who most idolize this nation, which in the midst of observators and astronomers could not produce a tolerable almanac, agree that we are superior to them. This confession perhaps is the effect of natural self-love. The Chinese form a nation entirely separated and different from us; whereas the antients are as it were of the same family with ourselves, and we regard them as our ancestors. And after all, some few sorry thousand miles can never be equivalent to a list of archons or consular Fasti. In short it is here, as in the compositions of the theatre, in which people suffer themselves to be much more easily deceived in what regards the customs and manners of the antient Greeks and Romans, than in those of the Turks, or Japonese.

Another instance in which this comparison holds good, between the antients and the moon at the horizon is, that she appears the greater to us upon the account of her being less resplendent there, than when she is at the meridian. Those objects which are the farthest off, are the least illuminated. So that if two objects, are of an equal size, the least illuminated will be thought the most distant, and consequently the biggest. Hence trees and houses appear greater to travellers in the twilight, than in full day; the sun seems bigger when seen through a cloud, and objects must generally appear greater in England, than they do

L

in Italy. The sun, after the death of Julius Cæsar, co[n]-
tinued pale and languid for the space of a year, and accor[d]-
ing to the expression of an elegant poet, threatened th[e]
guilty age with an eternal night. If the Romans h[ad]
dealt in observations, I do not doubt but they would ha[ve]
informed us, that he appeared likewise bigger than ord[i]-
nary. Objects then, said she, are magnified by the mi[st]
of antiquity: many of those great philosophers, who[se]
names now pass for a proverb, were perhaps no more [in]
their own time, than the regent of a college, or the le[c]-
tor of an university. Those, answered I, who are t[he]
most devoted to them, are the most likely to see them grea[t]-
ly magnified: for, as the finest and most judicious ver[se]
in the world inform us, fools *admire*, but men of *sen[se]*
approve; and every thing appears magnified to dulne[ss]
as objects do when seen through a mist. I should not [at]
all wonder, if some profound admirer of the Greeks shou[ld]
prefer the Epicurean explication of vision to that of t[he]
moderns, for this only reason, that one is more antie[nt]
than the other.

What explication is this, said the Marchioness, for I [do]
not remember that you have mentioned it to me before[.]
It was the last I spoke of, answered I, when we were tal[k]-
ing yesterday about the explications which the antien[ts]
have given of sight. This supposes that certain shadow[s]
or images fly off from bodies, by whose means we se[e.]
Though this may seem reasonable enough to some person[s,]
yet there arises a great difficulty to explain how it happen[s]
that when we are in the dark we see objects that are place[d]
in the light; but when we are in the light, we cannot di[s]-
cern objects placed in the dark: since according to th[e]
explication of the Epicureans in both cases, there are sh[a]-

ows which fly off from the objects, and raise in us the sensation of vision. Lucretius calls a certain lucid and subtile air to their assistance, which, entering into the eyes when they are in the dark, disengages them from the more thick and black air that obscured them, and by this means opens a passage to the shadows which from objects placed in the light proceed to the eye. When objects, on the contrary, are placed in the dark, the thick black air fills the eyes, and by this means, denies a passage to the shadows which are transmitted to the eye from those objects.

The image of any object, said the Marchioness, cannot be drawn upon the *retina*, unless there are rays transmitted from the object to the chrystalline humour, just as in the *camera obscura*, an object, in order to have its image painted upon the paper, must transmit rays to the *lens*. If then the object be placed in the light, and we in the dark, its image will be drawn upon the *retina*, and we shall discern it; but if the object be placed in the dark, it cannot transmit any rays to the chrystalline humour, there can be no image drawn upon the *retina*, and consequently the object cannot appear to our sight. But I do not see what relation there is between the thick or subtile air of Lucretius, and these images. It is true, answered I, that this air has nothing to do with the image on which vision depends, but it has a great relation to these shadows on which depends the *honour* of the Lucretian philosophy. And what is there in the world, that a philosopher, embarrassed in the explication of a phænomenon, does not lay hold on? But since you have so well explained this, I will venture to propose to you another, which you must often have observed; it is, that in going from a very light place to one which is much less so, and may even be cal-

led dark when compared with the other, the objects [of]
this place are at first not at all discernible, but by degre[es]
they begin to appear, and after some time are seen ve[ry]
distinctly. This often occasions great mistakes in societ[y,]
which are very soon found out, and repented of. A[s]
one, for instance, going into the chamber of a lady, wh[o]
either because she is indisposed or fancies herself to be [so,]
likes to sit in the dark, may take one person for anothe[r,]
and a fine compliment be wrong addressed, and the err[or]
afterwards appear to the great confusion of the person w[ho]
had been at so great an expence of wit in forming it.

This phænomenon, said the Marchioness, smiling, h[as]
very important consequences, and merits the utmost atten[-]
tion. But I must confess, it appears to me a little mo[re]
perplexed than the first, and I do not know how many de[-]
grees of subtilty in the air Lucretius would require to ex[-]
plain it by. Yet the explication of this phænomenon[,]
answered I, depends entirely upon a thing which you mu[st]
very often have observed with the utmost diligence. Hav[e]
you never remarked that there are no eyes, not even you[r]
own, but appear much finer by night than in the day? [I]
agree to this, said the Marchioness, that we may not spo[il]
our observations by compliments; But does it not procee[d]
from hence, that the night does not shew the defects o[f]
the face so much as the day, and therefor the eyes to[o]
must be gainers? The true reason of this phænomenon[,]
answered I, is, that in the dark, the pupil is more ope[n]
and dilated, which makes the eyes look blacker and bright[-]
er in the night than in the day, when the pupil is mor[e]
contracted. How many eyes have triumphed in the even[-]
ing and gained conquests which they lost the very nex[t]
morning at the approach of the sun! The pupil is contrac[-]

ed in very light places, in order that it may not admit too great a quantity of rays, which would only serve to do it hurt. On the contrary, it is dilated in the dark, enough to admit such a quantity of rays as are sufficient to cause vision. The reason perhaps, why some animals never creep out of their holes till evening is, because they are not able to contract their pupil so much as is necessary to hinder the light of the sun from injuring their eyes. When we go therefor from a light place, to one which may comparatively be called dark, the pupil, being at first very much contracted, does not admit such a quantity of rays into the eye, as is sufficient to raise the idea of vision. The pupil afterwards begins to dilate itself, and we begin to see. And as this dilatation is made by degrees, so we discern the object by degrees still clearer and clearer, till at last, when the pupil desists from dilating itself at a certain point, we afterwards continue to discern the objects with the same degrees of clearness.

You have not given me the least time to think on this, said she. Who can tell whether I might not have found out this explication, which now at least does not appear at all difficult to me? It is sufficient for you, Madam, said I, to have explained one phænomenon, and seen the difficulty of another. A very great exploit, truly, said the Marchioness with some emotion, to see difficulties and not be able to resolve them. It is a very great honour indeed for a general to besiege a town and not to take it! No, said I, but it is sometimes an honour for him not to undertake the siege at all. The first step to wisdom is to cease from folly, and the first point of learning not to be too arrogant, but perceive our own weakness. This is a point of modesty very little practised by those gentlemen who with the vulgar gain the reputation of philosophers, merely by the declaiming in assemblies and coffee-houses, against the antient philosophy which they know nothing of but the name, stigmatizing those who profess it with the title Ergotists, and having read perhaps some preface or literary journal. Such sort of persons never doubt of their knowlege, but explain and pass a decisive judgment upon every thing. These are blind men who would walk in a garden with the same freedom as other people, but the first bason they come to, fall in. There is an observation which the more it is examined, the truer it will appear, that nothing in the world is so difficult to be met with, as common sense.

I perceive, said the Marchioness, that I have some right to call myself a philosopher. I have my head full of vortices; I form light by the pressure alone of the globules of the second element, and colours by their rotation. have renounced the most agreeable qualities, and retain nothing but a little extension, and infinitely small quantities. I am not certain whether the world appears the same to all eyes: I explain one phænomenon, and see the difficulty at least of another; I think I have contempt enough for the antient philosophy; and after all this, I hope it will not be said that I am not wiser than I was. Do I want any thing else to make me a complete philosopher? — Yes, Madam, answered I, perhaps you should have a little less beauty, or make a better use of it. But you do not perceive that the philosophy you are so fond of needs a reformation, and I wish this reformation might be the last.

What, said she with some emotion, will you tell me that Vision is not performed in the manner you have hitherto explained it? This is plainly betraying me, and affirming upon your word, what afterwards appears not to be true. No, no, Madam, anſwered I, be not uneaſy, I am not of a character to propoſe to you things differently from what they are. Viſion ſhall remain untouched; that abjuration, which you have generouſly made of the roſes and lilies in your cheeks, ſhall ſtand good and be ratified in form. The doubts you are under, concerning the different appearance of objects in different perſons, ſhall ſtill continue to be reaſonable, and your preferring the moderns to the antients, ſhall ſtill be compatible, and remain as it is founded on the very beſt reaſons. The reformation I ſpoke of will affect nothing but the globules of light, and the manner in which they excite in us the ſenſation of colours. You may hereafter if you pleaſe regard the ſyſtem of vortices, as one of the fineſt and moſt entertaining philoſophical poems in the world, which is the idea under which I at firſt propoſed it to you. This is abſolutely diſconcerting my ideas, ſaid the Marchioneſs. I would willingly look upon this ſyſtem as ſomething more than a fable, were it ever ſo fine a one. I cannot think of changing any thing in the globules of light, which with ſo very little trouble ſupplied me with the moſt agreeable colours. If I once quit theſe, who knows how much pains, and how great an apparatus it will coſt me after this to make even a ſorry mezzotinto?

It will coſt you no more, anſwered I, than it did with your globules. This reformation was produced by father Malebranche; one of the greateſt and moſt illuſtrious Carteſians that ever appeared in the world. The authority of ſo great a name may let you ſee, how very neceſſary this reformation was, and you may moreover be ſure that the ſimplicity which has always formed the delight of this sect cannot fail here. This simplicity is an idol, to which they sacrifice every thing, even truth itself sometimes, that truth, which an antient called the citizen of heaven, and companion of the gods. But before I proceed to this reformation, it will be proper to lay before you the great difficulties which must make you for ever renounce your globules. This system, like Hercules in the fable, had very great difficulties to encounter with from its very birth; but perhaps it did not overcome them with equal honour.

Some objected, and with great reason, that according to those laws assigned to the vortices by their inventor himself, as the stars are not composed of the subtile matter, but of that of the third element, instead of being luminous, they would be covered with an opaque crust; and even if they were luminous, the contrary and equal pressure of the vortices would not suffer us to see them.

However weighty these objections might be, they would not be able to shake the faith of the steady Cartesians. But this, which I am now going to mention, appears an indissoluble gordian knot, even to the most zealous and ardent among them. You have this formidable enemy of the Cartesian philosophy in your own house, nay, in the very gallery where we are, and you do not perceive it. This painted wall is an adversary that makes war against the system you are fond of. Deliver me from this perplexity, I intreat you, said the Marchioness, or I shall erase the picture. You have a mind to make me quarrel with my own house for presenting me with such detestable objects. No, Madam, answered I, smiling, that is not my intention; I would rather have you persuaded that every corner of it is since yesterday become philosophical.

Let us fix upon one point in the air to which your eye

and mine may be equally directed while we are both looking at the same time upon different parts and different colours of this wall. Do you, for instance, place yourself at this pilaster, and look upon the red on the vesture of Achilles. I will stand at the window, and look upon the blue of the sea; so that while you are looking at the red and I the blue, our eyes may each be directed to the same point of air. It is certain, that two rays will pass through this point, one from the robe of Achilles, and the other from the sea. These rays you know are nothing but two series or strings of globules immediately touching each other, the one continued from the robe of Achilles to your eye, the other from the sea to mine. These two strings of globules intersect each other in that point which we have fixed in the air, and consequently in this point there will be one globule common to both strings. Do you understand all this? Yes, too well, said she, and I begin already to tremble. In order for these globules to excite vision in us, answered I, the pressure of those contained in that string, which comes from the robe of Achilles, must be continued from thence to your eye, and the pressure of those contained in that string which comes from the sea must from thence be continued to mine. Now that globule, which happens to be in the point of air, where the two strings intersect, and which is common to each of them, must at the same time press towards your eye and mine, which is utterly impossible if the globule be hard, as Des Cartes supposes it to be; because the close union of the parts of such a body can never suffer it to press at the same time towards two different sides. But this is not all. —— And yet this is sufficient, said the Marchioness, to demolish my globules. The very same globule, said I, as hard as it is, must have at the fame time two different rotations, one to excite in you the idea of a red colour, which is communicated to the whole ftring that comes from the robes of Achilles to your eye, and the other to excite in me the idea of an azure colour, communicated to the whole ftring that comes from the fea to my eye. But the difficulty will be ftill greater if we fuppofe other fpectators to be placed in this gallery, who all direct their eyes to the fame point in the air, as we have fixt upon, and other rays to pafs through this point, fome of which fhould convey the golden colour of Achilles's hair, that Minerva lays hold on in order to calm his deftructive and impetuous rage; others the green of this meadow, and the innumerable other colours which variegate the picture. You fee then, that fuppofing your globules, fuch as Des Cartes has made them, it would be impoffible for us to fee what, however, we really do fee. I underftand this but too well, anfwered fhe; but I befeech you, for the love of philofophy, never mention thefe globules to me again. I am refolved to think no more of them fince they have fo fhamefully yielded to the very firft difficulty. They feem to refemble thofe unexperienced lovers, who at the firft repulfe think of a retreat. But pray let me fee what your reformed Cartefian Malebranche fubftitutes in their place; for I am perfuaded he will be able to make a better refiftance.

Malebranche, anfwered I, entirely rejects thefe folid globules which you have forbid me to mention, and fubftitutes in their place certain exceeding fmall and fluid vortices compofed of an ethereal and very fubtile matter, which fills all the great vortices, as the great vortices which are the feats of ftars and light do the univerfe. Thefe little vortices, by that power which they have of dilating them elves, keep a mutual equilibrium in their respective vortices, just as the great vortices do in the universe. In this system of Malebranche, light is nothing but the undulation or vibration of the vortices, occasioned by the vibration of the luminous body which is always repelled in the same moment that it impels; and the greater or less force of the light depends upon the greater or less force of these vibrations, just as colour depends on their greater or less velocity. For instance, if these vortices should raise fifty vibrations upon the optic nerve of the retina, in any determinate space of time, it would give us the idea of a certain colour; if in the same time there should be a greater or less number of vibrations raised, we should have the sensation of a different colour. Malebranche ingenuously confesses however, that he was not able to assign what determinate degrees of quickness were necessary to form different colours in particular. A confession so much the more ingenuous as it is extraordinary in a philosopher.

This system of light and colours has a very great affinity with that of sound, with this difference only, that air is the vehicle or channel of the one, and ethereal matter or the vortices composed of that matter, the channel of the other. The vibrations, which a sonorous body when it is struck, raises in the air, and from thence in the auditory nerve, excite in us the idea of sound. In the same manner, the vibrations which a luminous body raises in the ethereal matter, and from thence in the optic nerve, excite in us the idea of light.

If the air be entirely excluded from any place, which may be done by the help of a certain machine, a sonorous body put into that place would not be heard to sound. In the same manner if it were possible to exclude the ethereal matter from any place, a luminous body put into that place would not appear refplendent.

The greater or lefs force of the vibrations on the air, or the auditory nerve, produces a great or lefs intenfenefs of found. In the fame manner the greater or lefs force of the vibrations on the ethereal matter, or the optic nerve, produces a greater or lefs intenfenefs of light.

The different quicknefs of the vibrations on the air, or the auditory nerve, produces different founds, as bafs, treble, and their different degrees; fo after the fame manner, the different quicknefs of the vibrations raifed in the ethereal matter or the optic nerve produce different colours, as red, yellow, and the like, which may be confidered as the tones of light.

I do not believe, faid the Marchionefs, that even our preachers ever carried a fimilitude farther than this. It may be carried ftill farther, anfwered I. As various and different vibrations crofs and interfect without deftroying, or rather, without giving each other the leaft interruption, which we every day fee in conforts of mufic, where the vibrations of the ftrings of a violin do not interupt thofe of any other inftrument, fo the different vibrations, which flow to our eye from different colours, do not interrupt each other, notwithftanding they crofs and interfect. The fluidity of thefe vortices gives them a power of tranfmitting the vibrations of different colours to various parts, which the folidity of the globules would not fuffer them to do; in the fame manner as the fluidity of the air does the different founds in a concert of mufic. The explication of this feems fo very difficult to Malebranche, that he affirmed a fyftem, capable of effecting it, muft be conformable to truth.

Sound and light, replied the Marchionefs, appear to be as faithfully copied from each other, as nature was by the paintings of Apelles, which were fo very accurately done, that an aftrologer could predict the future fortune of the perfons whom they reprefented.

I have not yet finifhed the comparifon, anfwered I. An object, placed between two looking glaffes over-againft each other, will be greatly multiplied. One candle is changed into a thoufand, and brings to mind the celebrated annual feaft of the illumination of candles among the Egyptians, from which, fome imagine the Chinefe to have borrowed their feaft of lanthorns. And does not the famous echo of the caftle of la Simonetta, not far from Milan, produce the very fame effect upon found? The report of a piftol in this place is repeated more than forty times, and a fingle inftrument of mufic forms a fulnefs of found fuperior to that of the moft numerous concert. Two great wings of a building oppofite to each other with windows, which are all falfe except one, and formed of a matter very proper to throw back the vibrations, reflect and multiply the found juft as the two glaffes do the candle.

The great lord Bacon, the harbinger of true philofophy, has among innumerable other curious things, propofed the examination of this affinity, betwixt light and found, to the confideration of naturalifts. Perhaps he could not have wifhed to find a more clofe union betwixt them, than what the fyftem of Malebranche difcovers. But he advifed too, that philofophers fhould carefully examine in what points they might difagree; and the greateft difference betwixt them is, as I firft told you, that the channel of found is the air, and that of light the ethereal matter. Hence it follows, that found muft be propagated from a sonorous body in time; for the spaces and interstices between the particles of air make it absolutely necessary, that there should be some little time before the motion can be communicated from one particle to another. Light on the contrary must be propagated in an instant, or an exceeding little space of time, because there are no spaces between the vortices or ethereal matter, since the whole universe is every where filled with them. Light and sound have the same resemblance to each other as the Nereids engraved by Vulcan upon the silver gates of the sun's palace, in Ovid's Metamorphoses. Their features are not exactly the same, but so extremely like, but it is very easy to perceive they are sisters.

Let us then become reformed Cartesians, said the Marchioness, by accepting a reformation which not only explains all that the globules did, but something more, and of much greater importance, which they were not able to explain. Let us adopt Malebranche's system of light and sound, these two new brothers in natural philosophy. I do not absolutely despair, answered I, but the harpsicord of colours, and the music of the eyes, which gives a still greater confirmation to this new alliance, may in time meet with a favourable reception from you.

What do you mean, replied the Marchioness, by this new invented music and harpsicord? Have you a mind to ridicule the philosophical similitude you have been entertaining me with? I should be sorry, answered I, to have any temptation to ridicule what you have adopted instead of your globules. This harpsicord is indeed a new invention, but is not therefor the less true or real. Upon moving the keys of this instrument, instead of hearing sounds, you will see colours and mezzotintos appear, which will

On LIGHT *and* COLOURS.

oduce the same harmony as sounds do. The sonatas of *Bononcini* or *Corelli* will give the same pleasure to the eyes when seen upon this philosophical harpsicord, as they do to the ear when they are played upon the common sort. The concords of a piece of purple and scarlet will raise the passions of love, pity, courage, or anger in our souls: This surprizing instrument is now making beyond the mountains, and you may for the future expect your silks and ribbons in music. The transient pleasures of the ear will be fixed in the eye; you may continually enjoy the fine airs of Farinelli wove in a piece of tapestry.

The inventor, answered she, probably took the first Idea of this, from the dress of a harlequin. However, we are greatly obliged to him, for we shall have no occasion to embarrass ourselves for the future in adjusting the colours of our clothes. We need only consult the thirds and octaves of this harpsicord, and we shall be sure never to make any discord in the shading. The painters, answered I, may find relief in their indispositions from this new invented music of colours, as singers and musicians are said to do from that of sounds.

Why will you restrain the effects of so singular a thing, said she, to the painters only? It will help physicians to increase their prescriptions and prolong their consultations. Physicians, answered I, must act with regard to their patients, as musicians do with weak voices; and as those are careful not to discourage their scholars with difficult notes, so these in certain distempers, as the bite of a tarantula, which can be cured only by pleasure, must take care not to prescribe any colours for which the patient has an aversion. But we must leave the physicians to divert their patients in this new method as they judge proper. This

M 2

new inftrument will help to give us a proof of the juftne[ss]
of that fine comparifon made by an elegant poet betwe[en]
the gradual languifhing and dying founds in the voice [of]
our tuneful Orpheus, and the infenfible fading and vanifh-
ing of the colours in the rainbow. Who knows, repli[ed]
the Marchionefs, but we may fome time or other form [a]
dinner by the affiftance of a harpficord, and find harmon[y]
in a fricaffee?

After this difcourfe, as we are taking the air in the garden, the Marchionefs fuddenly cried out,—What fhall w[e]
do! I fee a gentleman in the neighbourhood coming towards us, who in every vifit he makes does me the favou[r]
to repeat fonnets by the hundred, and yet always find[s]
time for fome ode. How fhall we difengage ourfelves from
his troublefome company? Will there be no vortex fo mer-
ciful as to fnatch him away with itfelf, and remove hi[m]
from our fyftem? For want of a vortex, anfwered I, w[e]
will ferve him as I once did a mathematician, who happened to be very talkative, a fault which thofe fort of people are feldom guilty of. When you are walking with [a]
friend, and difcourfing about the country of Kouli Kan, o[r]
fome fuch trifle, he will entertain you with the moft ab-
ftrufe points in geometry. He affaulted me one day as [I]
was walking with fome company in a garden, and w[e]
prefently found by his air, that he was preparing to torment us with his demonftrations and corollaries. I an[d]
the others who were with me began to talk of poetry
and repeat verfes, a language to which he was an utter
ftranger, without fuffering him once to open his mouth.
By this means we compaffed one of the moft difficult enterprizes, that of tiring the moft tirefome perfon in the world.
Now we need only continue our difcourfe upon philofophy,

and I will engage your sonnetteer will suffer the same punishment as my mathematician. Thus we resolved to proceed.

After the first compliments were over, the poet, who knew nothing of our scheme, took occasion to inform us, that the muses had for a long time used him ill, and that he was resolved to renounce them for ever. After we had civilly contradicted him, he answered, that he was ready to prove his assertion by a few sonnets which he had lately made, and which would shew us, how very little he was in their favour. If they are really so perverse, said the Marchioness, taking him at his word, you must entirely abandon, and never think of them again. We have just been discoursing on philosophy and optics; it will be taking an effectual revenge if you enter into our conversation, which is so very different from poetry. He excused himself by saying that he had not a capacity for such sublime objects, and though it was necessary sometimes to shew a little resentment, he must take care not to affront the muses too much. He observed that a little poetry would alleviate the severity of our philosophical discourses, and alleged the example and authority of Plato, who did not think it beneath him to write love-verses to Agatis, and engrave the three Graces on the citadel at Athens, with the same hand with which he had wrote the institutions of his Republic, and the Timeus, and in this manner divided his time between philosophy and the arts of Apollo. But all these arguments could not prevail on us to let him repeat his sonnets, which was the chief design both of his visits, and all that erudition which he had lavished upon us.

The Marchioness asked me several questions, which our poet did not think at all a-propos. Among the rest, she

was very anxious to know whether she might rely up[on]
Malebranche's system of light and colours, for the d[e]
struction of the globules made her fear every thing, a[nd]
her suspicions were terribly increased by this harpsico[rd.]
I answered, that such was the condition of all hum[an]
things, that nothing must hope for a long duration he[re]
below, a truth which our gentleman could evince by ma[ny]
fine verses of the best poets, and perhaps by some of h[is]
own. I added, that I was extremely pleased to find t[he]
example of the globules had warned her not to place t[oo]
much confidence in the reformation of father Malebranch[e.]
But that the most fatal blow to this opinion was, the b[e]
ing obliged to forsake it upon the account of that very an[a]
logy and correspondence betwixt light and sound, whic[h]
at first seemed to give it so much lustre.

This analogy, continued I, fails in one of the par[ts,]
and in that part where it was most wanted. And th[is]
circumstance is sufficient to overthrow Malebranche's r[e]
formed system. All those fine resemblances, which yo[u]
observed with so much admiration, cannot save it fro[m]
destruction.

If an undulating motion happens to meet with any ob[]
stacle in its way, this does not stop its progress, for i[t]
bends on all sides, and continues to propagate itself i[n]
spite of the obstacle that opposes it.

A very familiar example will make you understand wha[t]
I mean. If we were at the bottom of this hill, and som[e]
person on the opposite side of it should sound a French
horn to proclaim the destruction of some innocent tenan[t]
of the woods, whose only fault is the pleasure we find i[n]
destroying him by the help of our reason and contrivance[,]
we should hear this sound notwithstanding the whole hi[ll]

placed betwixt the horn and our ear. The reason of this is, because the undulations raised in the air by the french horn do not stop their progress when they meet with the hill, but giving way on every side and bending all round it, communicate the like vibrations to the opposite air. After the same manner, if you throw a little stone into this bason, the undulations formed in the water will not stop when they meet with the pipe, but giving way all round it, will communicate themselves indifferently to all the water, and thus the effects of it will be discovered in the whole bason.

You see then that if light were nothing but an undulation of the ethereal matter communicated to it by the vibrations of the lucid body, no interposed body could ever deprive us of the light of the sun or any other luminous object, or in other words, we should never have any shadow, which, especially in this season, would be a terrible inconvenience brought upon us by Malebranche's system. The pressure of Des Cartes' globules could give us no assistance in this case.

Thus Sir Isaac Newton, the avowed enemy of imginary systems, and to whom you are indebted for the true idea of philosophy, has at one blow lopped off the two principal heads of the reviving Cartesian Hydra.

Though the Marchioness perceived the force of this argument she did not seem greatly displeased with it. As she had renounced the globules, she easily gave up the vortices. But our sonnetteer was not quite so well satisfied. As he could find no opportunity of discharging his poetic fury, he was obliged to go some where else, to find an audience to a satire, which it is very probable he had begun to compose against philosophy.

DIALOGUE IV.

Encomium on Experimental Philosophy, and an Exposition of the NEWTONIAN *System of Optics.*

THE next day when we had disengaged ourselves from poetry, which had at first given birth to our discourses on light and colour, and afterwards endeavoured to disturb and interrupt it, I began after the following manner. It is now time, madam, to lead you into the most retired sanctuary of philosophy, from whence the prophane and those who are filled with vortices, globules, atoms, subtile matter, and like imaginations, are entirely excluded. This philosophy, which I am now conducting you to, is less pompous than that we have already discoursed on, but in return performs all its promises; a philosophy, which is contented with giving a history of physics, and leaves to others the province of making them the subject of a romance. You have had an instance of the one in its method of explaining the nature of vision, and the system of vortices has given you an example of the latter more pompous and splendid philosophy, which boldly goes to the first causes of things, and laying down certain arbitrary principles, upon these builds the world, and explains all the phænomena of it according to its own fancy.

As the eye is now discovered to have an entire resemblance to the artificial *camera obscura*, all philosophers will hereafter explain the nature of vision after the same manner. But there will not be that conformity in their opinions concerning the solidity of bodies, gravity, light, and colours, since the cause of these qualities can be known only by conjecture. And how very hazardous a thing this is, you have already seen in the Cartesian system of globules, to say nothing of Mallebranche's reformation, which, notwithstanding all the applauses at first given it, is now exploded, and shares the same fate as the globules. And this you may believe has been the case with all the general systems that have hitherto appeared, concerning the causes of things. They resemble vast empires, which totter and fall by their own weight and greatness. I find then, said the marchioness, that the *wherefore*, which so greatly excites our curiosity, will be for ever hid from us, and the pleasure of conjecturing, which is generally so adapted to the taste of men, will have no charms for philosophers. This really is a circumstance, which will make the condition of these gentlemen not greatly to be envied by the vulgar.

Conjecture, answered I, according to the assertion of one of the most ingenious authors in the world, is not to be allowed in any thing but geometry. In this science, if the certainty of principles does not directly guide us to what we seek, it never leads us however to any thing contrary, and always rewards our searches with somewhat equivalent. But what uncertainty and inconstancy is there in natural philosophy? Some affirm that there is a vacuum, or space void of all body, and others will have every thing to be body. This diversity of opinions, with regard to principles, must unavoidably produce very great and innumerable disputes as they advance further, which extend so far as the fixing the essence or nature of body, a thing which one would imagine should of all others be the mo[st] certain in physics, since body and the properties which d[e]pend on its essence, are the perpetual subject of philosoph[i]cal inquiries. I cannot help comparing these philosophe[rs] to those critical writers who correct some corrupted and d[e]fective passage of an ancient author. One of these gentl[e]men gives one reading, a second another, each supporte[d] with the finest and most elaborate arguments, and the en[]comiums of the journalists of the learned. Some old ma[]nuscript of the author at length appears drawn out from th[e] dust and obscurity of a library, and then all the fine read[]ings of these profound critics, and the time they spent i[n] inventing them, are sent into the regions of Ariosto's moon and are there treasured up among other lost things. Ob[]servations and experiment are the authentic and origina[l] manuscripts of nature; and these, by overthrowing so ma[]ny fine systems, instruct us every day to be more cautiou[s] in puzzling ourselves to form hypotheses. I look upon this advice as a very great benefit to mankind, since it ex[]empts them from no small trouble and fatigue. But the misfortune is, that men persist in a refusal of this friendly admonition, and are obstinately bent to spend their time to no purpose.

This is indeed a practice that redounds greatly to the honour of these observations of yours, said the marchioness. A system need only be ingenious, simple and elegant, to give them a right to declare open war against it. They may be termed the Erostratuses of natural philosophy, who found their glory in the destruction of all that is great and splendid. I must confess that I cannot be pleased with so malicious a character To what a height would your dis[]

a sure rise, answered I, if I had told you all that these
ervations are capable of effecting. There is perhaps no
tem better grounded than this, that animals have wings
en them in order to fly, and legs to walk. And yet ob-
vation has discovered to us certain insects who have large
ngs without making use of them to fly with; and in the
ne manner, there is one animal, which, notwithstanding
has legs disposed like that of others, formed in the same
anner and of the like proportions, yet almost always
alks upon its back with its legs upwards, just as if the first
re not sensible they had wings, nor the last, legs. It
true, however, that if observations had done no greater
vice to the world than to destroy, we should not be much
debted to them. But by overthrowing perplexed and
eless, and sometimes very troublesome systems, how ma-
good and useful discoveries have these observations fur-
hed us with, in the room of those hypotheses they have
erthrown?

Some melancholy philosophers have imagined the rays of
e moon were cold and humid, and therefor greatly to be
red, since there must be expected very dangerous effects
m their influence. And in fact you see many persons,
n now, who, believing the effects of this planet from the
dition of their fore-fathers, retire as soon as ever the moon
gins to rise, and, as they express it, gets strength; and
t numbers of people are persuaded that they have the
d-ach, if by walking in the evening they have unhappi-
been obliged to receive the infection of its light.

The experiments, which have been made upon this, give
full liberty to walk at what hour we please, without ap-
hending any danger from that quarter. The rays of this
net, collected in the focus of a burning glass or a lens, do

not cause any senfible effect in the bodies upon which t
fall, notwithftanding they are fometimes two thouf
times denfer when thus collected, than they ordinarily a
A thermometer, which is an inftrument containing a
quor that contracts with the leaft cold, and dilates w
the leaft heat, does not fuffer an alteration in the focu
thefe glaffes when they are expofed to the rays of the mo
whereas, if they are expofed to thofe of the fun, the
hemency of their heat furpaffes that of the hotteft furnac
fo that the *amiantus*, which defended the precious af
of antiquity from the devouring flames of the funeral p
cannot defend itfelf from the violent heat of thofe glaf
The rays of the moon do not appear to have any ot
quality, than that of fupplying the abfence of the fi
and infpiring a foft and pleafing melancholy in the hea
of lovers.

Thefe forts of obfervations, faid the Marchionefs, I ha
no objection to, which let the fine fyftems alone, and
liver mankind from ill-grounded fears. To this fp
of obfervation, anfwered I, we are indebted for our
liverance from other much more impotent fears; com
pillars of fire, fhowers of blood, and *ignes fatui*, ancien
marks of divine wrath, do not at prefent difturb fo mu
as one half hour's fleep, except it be in thofe perfons, w
will always be the vulgar, and always of a tempter fit
to receive thefe impreffions of terror from others.

But how much are we indebted to the ftudy of expe
ments! Aftronomy, natural hiftory, and anatomy, fe
by the affiftance of this to be rather new fciences born
mong the moderns, than tranfmitted from the antients
us. To this, anatomy owes the circulation of the blo
and all the animal œconomy, whofe very fimplicity was

g so little known among the antients. To
is obliged for its phosphorus: astronomy,
dictions: hydrostatics, for an easy method
arrying fresh air for respiration, in an ele-
) men: for acoustics, and their speaking
projects, for rendering the perfection of
to that of sight, and innumerable musical
e offspring of harmony. To this optics
copes, microscopes, magic lanterns, and
ber of other wonders, that perfect or flat-
seeing.

credulity, and a greater love for the mar-
ruth, negligence, and a want of proper
·vation, have for a long time been insuper-
) knowlege. How great a treasure of won-
il history, after having rejected the absur-
tients, demonstrated to us! New modes of
eathing, seeing and living, new conforma-
ew societies, new modes of being, unheard
o past ages.

of mankind has been polished in proportion
es has been more considered; and the arts
e been brought to perfection by observa-
in animals, commonly regarded either with
ie refuse of nature. Spiders have furnished
res with new species of silks; and the eggs
gh yet unknown, may, with a little appa-
a fine purple colour not inferior to that so
:d by the antients. Shall I inform you of
s made concerning the weight of air, and
s of dilating itself when compressed? expe-
rmed the wonders of Magdebourg. Shall

I give you an account of the equilibrium of fluids, vegetation and culture of plants, which have afforde[d so] great an advantage and ornament to fociety? By t[hese] experiments your garden is embellifhed with the pla[y] and agreeable murmur of artificial fountains; and t[hey] fupply the northern tables in great plenty with thofe [deli]cious fruits that nature had confined to a warmer he[mi]fphere. The orange, by thefe tranfported from Chin[a to] the Portuguefe foil, fweetly allays the burning heat of [the] fummer; and thefe experiments have extracted from [the] vines of the Rhine tranfplanted upon the burning rock [of] Canary, that agreeable juice fo pleafing to the tafte of [la]dies. Still better and better, faid the Marchionefs, [is] not this the clufter of the promifed land by which [you] hope to allure me? and as we are in the country, w[ould] intice me, by the hopes and advantages which accrue f[rom] obfervation, to agriculture and œconomy? Without [dif]pute you have thofe antient confuls in your head, [who] from the triumph returned to the culture of their farm[s.]

If I had a defign of inticing you, anfwered I, Mada[m,] I fhould rather entertain you with talking of the polite [arts,] of which you are fo fond, and which owe both their o[ri]ginal and progrefs to obfervation and imitation. Gr[ati]tude requires you to think yourfelf obliged to thefe for [the] pleafure you receive from the fine lineaments and eleg[ant] air of countenance in the Medufa of Strozzi, the juft g[ra]dation of the anger of Achilles, the variety and ftrength [of] paffions in Caffandra, that mafter-piece of the Timoth[eus] of our age, the majeftic folidity of the Portico of the R[o]tunda, the elegant ftrokes of Guido, and the magic [co]louring of Rubens. What riches has this induftrious p[hi]lofophy brought into the treafuries of painting, by t[he]

many new animals and plants? what an
has it given, by the imitation of the east-
ertain works defigned for the ufe of thofe
fuperfluity is neceffary? what a fruitful
and defcriptions has it by its new difco-
poetry? The fun, ftars, fhepherds, the
and the like common-place comparifons,
m the weight which they alone have long
and we from the fatigue of hearing them
l. How great a progrefs has the elegance
o greatly heightens the beauties of nature;
ie moft polite of all the arts, made in our
tance of a curious obfervation made upon
! beauty itfelf, the moft valuable treafure
ure can enrich and adorn youth, would
ind ufelefs gift, if obfervation had not con-
, by bringing in the ftrange, yet falutary
g ourfelves with a particular diftemper
leafe. How many fair Circaffians, who,
pleafure of the univerfe, are confined to
fubjected to the caprices of one fingle ty-
many beauties in England, the miftreffes
arts, owe their empires and their arms to
tion of the fmall pox?
ift on what you may poffibly think I might
it an advantage from, not to fay any thing
iral philofophy, which feems a province
d to the difcoveries of obfervations, is not
to *thefe* for that wife and real government,
he fouthern fun lefs pleafing than the cloudy
north, where the liberty of the people is
le with the authority of the fovereign?

Metaphysics, that labyrinth of reason, are obliged to th[em]
for a certain system of the origin and progress of our ide[as,]
and we for the knowlege of our selves. The chaos [of]
chronology and history has from these observations recei[v]ed its light and order. Sir Isaac Newton, that divi[ne]
philosopher, who may be regarded as the founder of h[u]man knowlege, has from observations drawn chiefly fro[m]
the ordinary course of nature, ranged historical facts in [a]
certain series, by joining epochas, which the ignorance [or]
pride of mankind had set at a great distance from ea[ch]
other, in the same manner as a judicious observation h[as]
united the boundaries of the earth in geography.

Conducted by this infallible guide, he, according [to]
the expression of one of his countrymen,

Display'd the lucid robe of day,

and thence extracted the true properties of light and c[o]lours, which had till that time lain concealed and involve[d,]
without forming, like Des Cartes and his followers, an
imaginary system to explain the nature of them.

This is a world entirely new, enriched with the most shin[-]
ing truths, and discovered by Newton alone; for there ar[e]
not the least traces of any philosopher who ever appeare[d]
there before him. His treatise of optics, the productio[n]
of thirty years study and search, is an excellent model [of]
true philosophy. One single experiment of his has ad[-]
vanced our discoveries more than all the ingenious an[d]
magnificent systems put together, that had ever gone be[-]
fore him.

An antique column of the most worthless stone has mor[e]
beauties in the eyes of a connoisseur, and will conduce mor[e]

to the perfection of architecture, than all the galleries of emerald and adamant, invented by the poets to adorn their inchanted palaces.

But your connoiſſeur, ſaid the Marchioneſs, cannot admire or taſte the beauties of a column, however antique and well-proportioned it may be, unleſs he firſt knows what a column is. And how is it poſſible that we ſhould underſtand the properties of light and colours, as you tell me Newton does, without firſt fixing what the colours themſelves are, and explaining the nature of them? Des Cartes, whoſe ſyſtem you moderns explode, tells me, that if a ray of light meets with the ſolid parts of a body, it is repelled and reflected, and I underſtand this very well, becauſe he had before told me that a ray of light is nothing but a ſtring of little globules. But how can I ever underſtand the new diſcoveries concerning the qualities of light, unleſs I am firſt informed what light itſelf is?

Is there any thing, anſwered I, more inexplicable than the nature and cauſes of muſcular motion? All the diſſertations of philoſophers upon it have been in vain. And indeed the more theſe diſpute upon the cauſes of things, the more inexplicable do they generally make them. And yet an excellent painter, a Michael Angelo, by laying down certain rules drawn from repeated obſervations, could have informed you, that when the body makes ſuch a particular motion or effort, certain muſcles muſt be elevated, and others lowered and depreſſed. So that there is no poſture ſo ſtrange but he could have foretold the various and almoſt infinite motions they could produce. The famous piece of the laſt judgment, in the Vatican, is an evident proof of his knowlege in this point.

The loadſtone is a ſecret of the ſame kind. Its nature

and the cause of its surprising effects are, and perhaps a[l]ways will be, as entirely lost to philosophers as the Pu[nic] language is to Critics.

Our ignorance of its cause, however, does not hinder [us] from making very many discoveries of its qualities. W[e] know, for instance, that if it be armed with steel it can a[t]tract a much greater quantity of iron than it can unarme[d]. We have discovered, that on one side it attracts anoth[er] loadstone, and repels it on the other, and constantly d[i]rects itself to the poles of the world. To this, natur[al] philosophy owes the discovery of a great number of truth[s], to this navigation its compass, and commerce and ma[n]kind very many advantages.

If it is ever possible to arrive at a knowlege of the natu[re] of things, this is the only method, by observing and i[n]vestigating, with the greatest attention, their most secr[et] and hidden properties, their primitive and elementary qu[a]lities, on which all the rest depend.

I observed to you the other day, answered I, that ever[y] ray of light, however slender, is nothing but a collectio[n] of innumerable other rays, which are not all of the sam[e] colour, notwithstanding the whole ray appears white[;] but some of these rays are red, orange, others yello[w], green, blue, indigo, or violet, besides innumerable d[e]grees of intermediate colours between each of these seve[n] principal ones. These rays of different colours, whic[h] are called *primary* or *homogeneal*, blended together for[m] a heterogeneous compound ray of a white or golden colou[r], such as a ray of the sun appears, just in the same manne[r] as different colours mixed together upon a painter's palle[t] compose a new one, which has something of all the othe[rs] in general, but is different from each of them in particula[r].

reasons why that poet, whom you disco-
rom his esteem for you, than by his stile, in
ht, uses the expression, *golden* and *sevenfold*,
tiently appropriated to the Nile, and the
es. This *sevenfold* light is the inexaustible
)se innumerable colours, which form the gay
: universe, and its rays are not tinged with
faphire, either when they are refracted
sm, or reflected from a surface, but derive
om the sun himself with that heat and lustre,
:ceive from him, though not discovered by

ery ray may be considered as a fibre composed
e other fibres or filaments, each of which
, a proper and unchangeable colour, which
ibly discover to our eyes, if it could be seen,
1 the other colours, which concur with it in
hite or yellowish colour of light. But how
must be the industry of that philosopher,
ide and resolve the whole ray into its pri-
entary rays, so that every one of them should
colour? It is certain this division could ne-
these primary and homogeneal rays were
nature that some are refracted more than
ing all with the same inclination out of one
another, from air into glass, for example,
eans are disunited and separated from each

ition, that *rays which differ in colour differ
of refrangibility*, is the fundamental disco-
iich the Newtonian system of optics is built.
his it is demonstrated that the violet rays are

the moſt refrangible of all. Next follow the indigo, then the blue, green, yellow, orange, and laſtly the red, which are the leaſt broken of any by refraction. Do I explain myſelf clearly enough, Madam, for you to conceive my meaning?

Extremely well, anſwered ſhe: I underſtand very eaſily, that nature, by making rays which are different in colour different likewiſe in refrangibility, has furniſhed philoſophers with a means of ſeparating them, which otherwiſe would be impoſſible. The properties of this light, which you have been deſcribing, are indeed very ſurprizing. A philoſopher muſt have a very great and enterprizing genius that could make ſuch diſcoveries; and his credit ought to be ſupported by very weighty arguments drawn from frequent obſervations, which I muſt confeſs I am extremely impatient to be acquainted with. I who was at firſt a Carteſian, afterwards a diſciple of Malebranche, now find myſelf without any ſyſtem at all. This is a vacuum that does not greatly pleaſe me, therefor I am in haſte for it to be repleniſhed with other obſervations.

Theſe will very ſoon amply repair the loſſes you have ſuſtained by them, anſwered I. It would be well if every thing elſe in the world, that does us an injury, would make as good a compenſation for it.

Imagine yourſelf to be in a place of Milton's viſible darkneſs, or rather ſtill darker a place, if you will be abſolutely deprived of all light; and this ſhall be our theatre of reaſoning and obſervations.

Let a ray of the ſun enter in at a hole made in the window ſhutter, and let a glaſs priſm be placed horizontally at this hole, to refract the ray in ſuch a manner as to throw it upon a wall oppoſite to the window, ſo that as it is going out of the priſm, it is almoſt horizontal and parallel to the pavement of the chamber; whereas if it had not been refracted, but direct, it would fall upon the pavement itself, and there form a white image of the sun of a figure almost round. That spectrum, or image of the sun, which the refracted ray forms upon the wall, is very different from that which the direct ray formed upon the pavement; for as the image of the direct ray was almost round and entirely white, that of the refracted ray is of a figure nearly resembling a fish at cards, and varied with an infinite number of colours, among which the seven primary ones are distinguished and placed in a shining order, one after another.

The jolly peacock spreads not half so fair
The eyed feathers of his pompous train;
Nor golden IRIS *so bends in the air,*
Her twenty-colour'd bow through clouds of rain.

FAIRFAX.

I am very glad to find that Tasso, said the Marchioness, who had before a little transgressed against the laws of refraction for the sake of his Armida, has amended his fault, and is at present reconciled to optics.

These colours, answered I, with which the image is painted, are disposed in such a manner, that the red is in its lower extremity; above this is placed the orange, afterwards the yellow, then the green, the blue, indigo, and lastly the violet, which is placed in the upper part of the image. Innumerable degrees of intermediate colours insensibly connect and unite the same primary ones. Neither Correggio, Titian, nor his rival Rosalba, did ever unite and shade their mezzo tinto's with so much exactness to form the oval of a face.

In order to explain this great change, we must suppose

one of thefe two cafes, either that light is compofed of rays differently coloured and differently refrangible, fo that the prifm does nothing but feparate them from each other, when they are tranfmitted through it; and by this means the different colours are formed, and the image which would otherwife be round, is of an oblong figure: this is one manner of explaining this phænomenon. The other is, that the light in paffing through a prifm, acquires colours which it had not before, and moreover, that every ray is fhattered, dilated, and fplit into many other diverging rays painted of a different colour; and this is the reafon why the image is coloured, and of an oblong figure.

This laft is the fuppofition of Grimaldo, a philofopher, who preceded Sir Ifaac Newton; and this fyftem is called the *difperfion* of light. You fee it is neceffary, unlefs we admit the different refrangibility, to fuppofe this difperfion, in order to explain why the coloured image of the fun fhould have a length much greater than its breadth, after being refracted by the prifm.

This experiment, faid the Marchionefs, which has coft me fo much attention to underftand, and this oblongitude of the folar image, are not fufficient to prove the different refrangibility, becaufe all this phænomenon may be as well explained by Grimaldo's difperfion of the light, which is a fyftem very different from Sir Ifaac Newton's. I want to fee fome experiment which cannot poffibly be explained by any other fyftem than the Newtonian, and that I believe would fatisfy me. This, anfwered I, is the very thing neceffary to prove not only the different refrangibility, but every other principle in philofophy; and this, Sir Ifaac Newton has done, without knowing, perhaps, that it would one day give pleafure to

hatever a certain author may say to the con-
:cuses him with having drawn more conse-
his observations than he ought to have done,
reatest faults that a mathematician can be
. This author reproaches Sir Isaac, with
:d the different refrangibility of the solar rays
:eeding observations; whereas Sir Isaac de-
efs terms, that the observation is not suffici-
purpose, because this strange appearance of
ay proceed from the shattering of the rays,
supposes; or from an inequality of refracti-
tant, but only casual, and therefor can have
ced from it. The more scrupulous this great
appears in his reasons, the more licentious
rsary seem in his accusation. In order to re-
persion of Grimaldo, and the fortuitous ine-
e refractions, he invented the following ex-
iich is, as it were, the arbitrator and judge
versy.
d the coloured image formed by the prism,
n the wall, upon the face of another prism
ht in such a manner, that the red of the image
pon the lower, and the violet in the superior
ice, and the other intermediate colours should
:ly in the intermediate spaces betwixt the red
t.
t prism, which was placed horizontally, re-
rays upwards, this second, placed upright,
them sideways, either on the right or the
if they were at first thrown almost directly
ll opposite to the window, they must now
ue, and with some inclination. The refrac-

tion then which the colours are to fuffer in paffing fide ways through this fecond upright prifm, is the thing whic[h] muft determine the queftion, either in favour of Sir Ifaa[c] Newton's fuppofition of the different refrangibility, or f[o] Grimaldo's notion of the fhattering of the rays, or laftl[y] muft give the preference to a fortuitous and cafual ine[quality] quality of the refractions, which cannot agree with an[y] fyftem at all. For, if the folar image, formed by the fir[ft] prifm which refracted the rays upwards, received its c[o]lour and oblong figure from a difperfion or dilatation [of] every incident rays, a fecond tranfverfe and fideways re[fraction, caufed by the fecond prifm, muft after the fam[e] manner fhatter and dilate the rays of this image fideway[s] and render it of the fame oblongitude in breadth as it ha[d] before been in length; fo that a new image would b[e] painted upon the wall of the chamber, which is behin[d] the fecond prifm; and this image would be coloured di[f]ferently from what it was before, and be changed fro[m] an oblong figure, to one almoft fquare.

Laftly, if the colours and oblong figure of the imag[e] formed by the firft prifm, were occafioned by a fortuitou[s] and accidental inequality of refractions, who can tell wha[t] variations chance might have produced in the combinatio[n] of the fecond prifm, and in the new refraction which tha[t] prifm gave to the light?

Whatever effects chance might produce in this cafe, i[t] is certain it could never agree with what the Newtonia[n] fyftem aims at. According to this fyftem, if the colourin[g] and oblong figure of the image formed by the firft prifm were occafioned by the feparation of rays differently co[]loured and differently refrangible, a fecond refractio[n] made fideways, can only incline this image, and mu[ft]

same as it was before with regard to its
ong figure.

incline the image, said the Marchioness?
stand the reason of this. You will soon
answered I, when you reflect, that if the
as removed, the rays would all strike the
a direct line. Now if the second prism re-
t rays, that is, turns them sideways and
of their path, more than it does the red,
ce the wall more oblique than these, or in
le violet must fall at a greater distance from
the red. The intermediate colours too,
d and the violet, will fall upon intermediate
all: thus the image will appear inclined,
eaning with its violet extremity farther from
the red is. These effects must happen ac-
Isaac Newton's system; and these in reality
I myself have often had the pleasure of see-

second prism, there be placed a third and
r that the image may be successively refrac-
hrough them all: those rays which were
than the rest in the first prism, will be more
the following prisms. But the image will
deways, nor coloured differently from what

he Marchioness, has pronounced the grand
of three systems that contended for it, the
carried the golden apple. I must confess
es not displease me; for to say nothing of
inequality of refractions, which does not
e, Grimaldo's supposition of the shattering

O

and dilatation of every particular ray, had something t[oo]
perplexed and imbarraffing in it. If you think the jud[ge]
ment which nature has pronounced in favour of our ph[i]
lofopher, anfwered I, to be fo juft, that of his adverfar[y]
whom I lately mentioned, will appear extremely capri[ti]
ous, who afferts, that Sir Isaac Newton has, by agreeab[le]
experiments, confirmed the obfervations of Grimaldo. [I]
am not fo greatly furprized at this adverfary, replied t[he]
Marchionefs, who does not appear to have any great know[-]
lege of the matter, as at Grimaldo himfelf, who negle[c]
ted to prove the truth of his difperfion of the rays, by
eafy and fimple an experiment as this, which requires n[o]
thing more than a fecond prifm after the firft. One woul[d]
imagine, that it fhould have been very obvious to a pe[r]
fon bent upon making a fyftem. Say rather, anfwered
to a perfon long exercifed in the arts of obfervation; for
love of building fyftems, and making experiments, are tw[o]
things that feldom go together. But it generally happer[s]
that the moft fimple things are the moft difficult, and cor[n]
fequently the longeft before they are found out. Th[e]
circulation of the blood, for example, appears to be
very eafy difcovery, and one would imagine fhould hav[e]
been very antiently made. When an orifice is opened i[n]
the arm, the arteries fwell from the heart towards the ex[-]
tremities of the body, and the veins, on the contrar[y]
from the extremities of the body towards the heart. Thi[s]
evidently fhews, that certain veffels, that is, the arterie[s]
are defigned to convey the blood from the heart to th[e]
extreme parts, and other veffels, namely the veins, to car[-]
ry it from the extremities to the heart. Befides, the deat[h]
of Seneca might have furnifhed the antients with a phy[-]
fical experiment, as well as a moral precept. It was im[-]

possible that all the blood should be emitted through the opening of the veins, unless those of the superior parts had communication with those of the inferior; or in other words, unless it circulated through the whole body. It appears then that it was much easier for the antients to discover the circulation of the blood, who had so many experiments ready prepared to their hands, than for Grimaldo to find the falshood of his dispersion, because his experiments must have been the effect of his own labour and invention.

It is true, some bigots for antiquity pretend to find this discovery in Hippocrates, so that according to them, all the inventions of the moderns, and all our distempers, were known to the antients. But this notion is the same as if a Vellutellus, or some other zealous admirer of Petrarch, should discover the Newtonian system of optics in these verses,

While the great author of his frame expires,
The conscious sun withdraws his active fires;
Pale sickly shades ov'rspread his languid ray,
And ev'ry beauteous colour fades away.

The most simple things are generally discovered the latest, and with the greatest difficulty. This aphorism, said the Marchioness, is too well verified even in the toilet, where an elegant, but simple disposition of our hair, or our patches, often costs great trouble, and the utmost anxiety of mind.

According to this principle, answered I, Sir Isaac Newton's experiments must have cost him an infinite deal of labour. For if the preceding experiment, to prove the different refrangibility of the rays, is at once simple, a greeable, and conclusive, all the others which he invente for the same purpose, are no less perfect, and yet appe so very obvious, that every one would imagine he himse might have as easily found out.

How, said the Marchioness, is not this experiment suff cient to prove the different refrangibility without seekin for any more? Have I acted wrong, in suffering myself t be too easily convinced? No, Madam, answered I, a lad cannot err in this point. But Sir Isaac Newton himse does not desire you should assent to his system so foo This experiment, without dispute, is sufficient to demor strate the different refrangibility, but not to satisfy a ph losopher resolved to try nature a thousand ways, and pu her to a thousand proofs, in order to establish his belief o a sure foundation. You seem, said the Marchioness, t represent nature as a coquet, and Sir Isaac Newton as jealous lover, who never thinks he has proof enough c the fidelity of his mistress. This, however, answered I was the only object of his love. I am very sorry, that cannot shew you all the experiments which he invented fo this purpose, in order to present you with the most finishec and beautiful piece that philosophical jealousy ever com posed. But the parts I shall shew you will assist you to form an idea of the whole, just as the obelisks and amphithea tres discover the grandeur of antient Rome. Let me in treat you, said the Marchioness, to make me a complet Newtonian. I plainly see that by my conversion I shal acquire the knowlege of truth without losing that pleasure which I found in being deceived.

In the dark chamber which we have prepared for ou experiment, continued I, let a white thread be extende horizontally against the window, but at some little distance from it. Let two rays of the sun enter at two holes made in the window-shutter, which, refracted by the two prisms, may paint two coloured images upon the opposite wall. When this is done, we must recommend ourselves to the genius which presides over optics, and then patiently wait till the half of this thread be illuminated by the red rays of one image, and half of it by the violet rays of the other. Let the wall opposite to the window be covered with a black cloth, that the colours which would otherways be reflected by the wall, may not disturb the experiment; for at present we want no other colours but those of the thread, which must be alone distinguished. This thread must be observed through a prism placed before the eyes in such a position, that all the objects seen through it appear higher than they really are. The thread too will appear to be transported higher by the refraction; but because the violet half should suffer a greater refraction than the red, it will be much more transposed than the red, so that the thread will appear divided into two parts, the one illuminated with violet, the other with red, and the red will appear lower than the violet.

This experiment, if we should exclude every other, is intirely agreeable in its parts to the Newtonian system. If the violet part of the thread be illuminated with indigo, the thread will appear less divided than at first, the indigo half approaching nearer to the red than the violet did, which must necessarily happen, because the difference of refrangibility between the indigo rays and the red, is less than that between the red and the violet.

If from indigo this half be illuminated with blue, the other half still remaining red, the thread will, for the same reason as I before mentioned, appear less divided than first, and still successively less if it be illuminated with the other colours in order, green, yellow, and orange, till length becoming red like the other half, the thread will no longer appear broken nor divided in two as at first, but whole and continued, because now the colours of each half have no difference in their refrangibility.

A like experiment may be made with a paper, the one half coloured with red, and the other blue; placed afterwards upon a black cloth, and looked at through a prism it will appear broken and divided into two parts. A paper illuminated with four colours, which I have myself seen demonstrated, that is, red, yellow, green and blew ranged one after another in the order I have named them appeared through a prism divided into four pieces, like the steps of a ladder. The blue is sometimes the highest of all, and sometimes lowest, as the position of the prism requires. This experiment varied in as many ways as the fruitful imagination of Paul Veronese would vary the subject of a picture, always succeeded so well, as to have greatly confirmed this system, if its author suffered it to need any confirmation.

I must ingenuously confess, said the Marchioness, that though I have always regarded the mathematicians with a singular veneration, I do not yet understand what their demonstrations are. However familiar they may at present be rendered, I do not comprehend them enough to find the solution of a problem among the patch-boxes and perfumes on my toilette. I now begin to fear that my ignorance of the Deity I worshipped, greatly increased my veneration for it. Their evidence causes so great a noise in the world, that I was persuaded every thing else, however well it might be proved, had only a small degree of probability when compared with these. At present, I cannot conceive it possible for any mathematical demonstration to be more certain than Sir Isaac Newton's different refrangibility, and yet this is a thing merely physical. But you are to consider, Madam, that the person, who has treated upon this physical subject, was the greatest mathematician that ever appeared in the world. We may affirm then, replied the Marchioness, that as every thing which Midas touched was transformed to gold, so every thing that Sir Isaac Newton handled became demonstration.

If ever physics could hope to vye in certainty with geometry, answered I, they might with some reason expect it, when treated by Sir Isaac Newton, though there is a a very great difference in the nature of their proofs.

Physics can only consider a vast number of particulars, make observations upon them, and thence deduce general propositions; whereas geometry, by a more expeditious and certain way, abstracts particular cases, and founds its demonstrations upon nature; and the idea of the thing itself, whereon it treats.

All that a mathematician demonstrates to you concerning one triangle, will be true in all, be they of what species they will, because he considers nothing but what is necessarily included in the nature of a figure terminated by three right lines; and as this is found in all triangles that can possibly be either made or imagined, his proposition will hold true in all.

On the other hand, a naturalist will tell you, that all bodies here below gravitate, and if left to themselves descend; but he does not, like the mathematician, deduce this proposition from the nature of body, for that is unknown to him, but from a daily obfervation that gold, filver, gems, water, air, and a thoufand other bodies gravitate, and do it conftantly by day and night, in fummer and winter, fair and cloudy weather; from whence it may reafonably be inferred by induction, that every other body gravitates at all times, and in all places.

But however reafonable this method may feem, fo great a demand for proofs implies a want of demonftration, juft as a too great attention to drefs, argues fome defect of natural beauty in a face. Who can tell, but notwithftanding fuch a multiplicity of obfervations, fome may queftion whether there be not a certain body with which we are yet unacquainted, that has no gravitation ? or if there be not fome country in the unknown tracts of the fouthern pole, where bodies have not that quality of gravitation which we difcover them to be endowed with in all the known world ? Or laftly, whether in paft ages there may not have exifted a certain body that did not gravitate ? You will grant, however, faid the Marchionefs, that where the number of obfervations is fo great as that from whence the gravitations of bodies, and the different refrangibility of the rays of light are deduced, that perfon muft be inexcufable who doubts their evidence, unlefs it was prefcribed him by a phyfician for his health.

If there are fome, anfwered I, too exceffive in their doubts, there are many others too bold in their affertions. All do not imitate the prudent and neceffary referve of our judicious philofopher : fome are contented with one fingle particular cafe, from which they haftily deduce a general conclufion, like thofe who form a judgment of the temper and general character of a whole nation, from the particular humour of a single person, whom they have seen perhaps once or twice at a coffee house.

Sir Isaac Newton's antagonist whom I lately mentioned, imagining he had overthrown the system, and principally the different refrangibility, in order to prove himself the opponent of this great author, even in the method of philosophifing, has put together a general system, hinted at by others but not followed, formed upon particular cases, which, well examined, are nothing but consequences of that which he imagined himself to have overthrown. He supposes certain grounds, and a mixture of light and shade; and the different combinations of these are, according to his opinion, the cause of different colours.——Can a combination of light and shade, interrupted the Marchioness, ever produce red or yellow? A phænomenon must be very unfortunate, whose explication depends on this system. Perhaps, answered I, those phænomena which contradict general laws, those monsters of optics, if there are any such, are sent by nature to this system for their explication; and do not these fine colours of yours too deserve a little punishment for all the mischiefs they have caused? But see the unhappy condition of the poor prismatic colours, which certainly do not merit the correction that yours do; and from hence you may form an idea of the value of this system.

It affirms, that when a ray of the sun is refracted by a prism, these colours are produced by means of two sorts of images; the one formed by the dispersion of the solar rays, and the other, by that of the rays of heaven, which are contiguous to those of the sun. What, said the Marchioness, does this philosopher attempt to bring this *dispersion* again upon the stage? Had he never seen the experiment of the second upright prism, which has for ever banished this supposition from the province of optics?

Authors, answered I, have their eyes formed differently from those of other men. The sun is light, and the sky comparatively dark. This was sufficient to furnish the philosopher we are speaking of, with abundance of relations betwixt light and shade, the veils, as he expresses it, formed by these two images, from whence he draws an explication of the difference of colours in a prism. I fancy, said the Marchioness, this explication will not be very simple; it appears to me sufficiently perplexed. Not to insist upon this and many other difficulties which this system is chargeable with, we will confine ourselves to the following objection, answered I.

If it be true that this diversity of colours depends on a mixture of the rays of these two images of the sun and sky, and from their shaddowing each other, it is certain that if there can be found a method to prevent the celestial rays from coming to the prism, and consequently from being refracted and mixt with those of the sun, the colours will vanish with all that fine theory which arises from the mixture of those two sorts of rays.

Now this may easily be effected, if before the ray of the sun, which enters at the window of the dark room, be refracted by the prism, the middle of the ray be transmitted through another hole made in a table, or a pastboard placed at some distance from the window: In this case, so far is the prism from receiving the celestial rays contiguous to those of the sun, that it receives no rays from the sun himself, but what flow from his disk, and is not at all affected by those that proceed from his edge. It is evident then, that if this system be true, the colours of the

cafe could not appear, which is abfolutely
perience, a difgrace pretty familiar to this

faid the Marchionefs, to refemble Bacchus
n the giants, who attempted to dethrone
rder to ufurp their places. The fpirit of
:ars no lefs ftrong in this author, than in
tuous fons of earth.

fuppofe, anfwered I, that an author is often
fircus of giving his name to a new fyftem,
idy can be of giving her's to a new fafhion.
ould they be, if, like that Chinefe emperor,
l the books of hiftory preceding his reign, in
:e his name the firft epocha of it, they could
:ceding fyftems to make their own the epocha
owlege!

r Ifaac Newton's fyftem came from a country
d the Alps, to be favourably received among

It would be very furprizing, if a fyftem,
England, had not been treated with averfion
ms in a country fo near the fun as ours. I do
ed the Marchionefs, why a fyftem fhould meet
fe ufage for being a native of England. For
much an Italian as I am, I do not believe
be prejudiced againft a well-grounded one,
id been produced in Ireland, or Nova Zem-

not to imagine yourfelf, anfwered I, to be
the generality of mankind. A fea, a river, or
nountains placed between fome people and a
i, are infuperable objections to their reception
ips as the Romans found a certain *Je ne fçais*

quoi, in the ſtile of Livy, which diſcovered the *Paduan*, ſo our Italians find a *Je ne ſçais quoi*, in every truth tha[t] comes from beyond the Alps, which does not agree wit[h] their taſte. Theſe gentlemen, ſaid the Marchioneſs, mu[ſt] have a very diſtinguiſhing judgment to diſcover ſuch di[f]ferences as theſe, or it rather argues, they have no taſt[e] for truth, who find any thing foreign in the proofs of different refrangibility. In this I may venture to affir[m] myſelf a better Italian than they, ſince the leaſt differenc[e] in this caſe may turn to our diſadvantage.

You, Madam, ſaid I, are a citizen of the world, and you[r] ſenſes formed for truth are proof againſt the objections o[f] thoſe who only appear to be zealous for it. You will find a nev[v] demonſtration of the different refrangibilities drawn from th[e] difference in the focus of a lens, through which the differen[t] colours are viewed. The image of the letters of a book formed by a convex glaſs, illuminated by the red rays o[f] a priſm, appears diſtinct at a certain diſtance from th[e] glaſs: the image of the ſame letters, when illuminated b[y] the blue rays, is not diſtinct, but at a leſs diſtance. I[n] the like manner, the four colours, red, yellow, green, and blue, of the paper we before mentioned, are not equally diſtinct when placed at an equal diſtance from the lens. The blue is neareſt, next follows the green, afterwards the yellow, and laſt of all the red, whoſe rays being leſs refrangible than the reſt, muſt be collected and united at a greater diſtance from the lens.

Might not ſome wiſe caviller, ſaid the Marchioneſs ſmiling, gravely object, that the book which firſt received the red, and afterwards the blue rays, was wrote in Engliſh; and that in order to prove the different refrangibility, it was neceſſary for it to be Italian? But after all, it is an in-

On LIGHT and COLOURS.

mous thing to be so hardened against truth. Are not these experiments sufficiently decisive? And can there in any country of the world be assigned a cause, why the image of one colour should be nearer to a lens than that of another, unless it be the different refraction which they suffer in passing through the lens? Do not put yourself in a passion, Madam, said I; the different refrangibility will be true, notwithstanding these objections. You may still safely believe it, as many other judicious persons do, in defiance of that obstinate war which the antagonist of our philosopher declared against it. The Newtonian system had the same fortune as that field where Hannibal encamped when he besieged Rome, which did not sell at all the worse upon that account: or rather, you may look upon these objections, as the satirical verses, those miserable invectives which the licentiousness and malignity of the common soldiers mixt with the acclamations and glory of a Roman triumph. The beauty and simplicity of this system did not deserve to pass unmolested by envy and censure, that tax which merit is bound to pay to the public.

A celebrated minister * at once capable of the sublimest projects and the lowest employments, and a whole college, joined their forces against the applauses paid to the Cid. For a like reason, Moliere's Misanthrope was recited to the same audience that listened to the sermons of Cotin. How often have the celebrated Coracci had the mortification of seeing their fine pieces sold in their life-time by the ll, if I may use that expression, which now are the ornaments of the best chosen galleries, and paid by the ad-

---

* Cardinal Richelieu.

P

miration of connoisseurs, better than by the gold of t[he]
rich!

It was necessary for the honour of Sir Isaac Newto[n's]
system, that it should be attacked on all sides, and th[at]
some should dispute the different refrangibility of the ra[ys,]
while others wrangle about the immutability of colou[r,]
which is another of their properties discovered by our p[e]-
netrating philosopher.

The experiment, upon which this new quality of colou[r]
is principally founded, was renewed in France, by mo[n]-
sieur Mariotte, a man exceedingly well versed in the ar[t]
of observation. This experiment in his hands produced a[n]
effect contrary to what Sir Isaac Newton had given reaso[n]
to hope for. Thus a system, the slow and considerat[e]
offspring of reason and experience, was esteemed imagi[-]
nary and vain; and a great philosopher, who spent hi[s]
whole life in the study of truth, passed for a reveur, or a[n]
impostor.

What is this you tell me, said the Marchioness, of a[n]
experiment in France contrary to that of Sir Isaac Newton[?]
Is it possible, that two men equally attentive, and accu[s]-
stomed to observation, should need a third to decide [a]
matter of fact? It is not surprising that two people shoul[d]
reason differently upon the circumstances of a fact accord[-]
ing to their different principles, as in the case of a person,
who shifted his linen three times a day, one asserted that
he must be extremely neat, and the other, that he was [a]
very sloven. But to dispute and mutually deny the fact
itself, I always thought reserved for silly women and en-
thusiasts.

It is certainly, answered I, a great reflection upon philosophers, when we find them dissent in matters like these;

at least demonstrates, that one of them must have been inattentive in observing the laws of nature. Those rational horses so far superior to us men, which Gulliver discovered in the island of the Houyhuynms, the last place where he arrived at in his allegorical voyages, were extremely surprized to find such contradictions among our philosophers, that is, those of our species who take the most pains to cultivate their reason. Those happy animals know not the meaning of uncertainty and doubt, in matters of fact. The dishonour that philosophers receive upon this account is very great, even among us, and there are too many examples of it.

Two famous academies, which have equally truth for their end, and emulation for their companion and guide, disputed upon a fact, by which is demonstrated the refraction which light suffers in passing from a vacuum into air. That academy, which maintained the refraction, was at length victorious; and it was necessary that even this truth should be contested in order to be admitted. Some from experience will tell you, that in breathing, the air passes from the lungs to the heart, while others allege the same experiment to prove that it does not. Many discover certain little machines and organizations in the glands of a body, which others affirm cannot be seen. Fancy and prepossession have the same influence here as in all other things, and make us think we discover in objects, without us, what runs strongest in our own mind. Thus a few irregular strokes will appear to the eyes of a painter, the contour of a leg or a face, wind-mills become giants to Don Quixot, and fires and beeches seem transformed to a fine lady in the eyes of a lover.

An observer must not search into experiments, in order to find his own opinions there, like that perfon w[ho] looked for his pedigree in Homer, becaufe both the o[ne] and the other will every where meet their own imagina[ti] ons. Natural philofophy, like poetry, requires a m[an] formed exprefsly for it, a Malpighi, a Reaumur, a Boyl[e,] not moved by authority, feduced by fancy, nor terrifi[ed] by difficulties; a man, if we will believe a celebrated write[r,] dexterous, active, and curious as the French and Englifl[h] and referved, cautious and circumfpect as the Italians an[d] Spaniards. Why not the patience of fome other natio[n,] faid the Marchionefs, inftead of the caution of ours, whic[h] is too like diffidence to redound greatly to our honou[r.] This author, anfwered I, confiders only the good qualitie[s] of different nations. But you would be better pleafed perhaps, if the part we contribute to the formation of [a] perfect philofopher, were the religious attention of ou[r] paffionate lovers. I am acquainted with one of thefe, fai[d] the Marchionefs, who would be a Newtonian if philofoph[y] was his miftrefs.

This attention, anfwered I, might carry thefe gentlemen to a great height of fuperftition, as it does a naturalift, who prefcribes it as a rule of art, whenever an experiment is made, to mark exactly the country, hour of the day in which it was effected, what wind blew at that time, the degree of heat, and draught of the air, with many other circumftances of this nature, which in fome cafes may be proper, and even abfolutely neceffary, but in others I really do not fee of what fervice they are; for in looking upon a paper of two colours with a prifm, it is of no fort of importance whether the wind blows eaft or weft, whether the time of the year be autumn or fpring, the feventh or twentieth day of the month. Thefe circumftantial na-

...uralists resemble an antiquarian, who should copy a cornice of an inscription with as much exactness as the inscription itself.

Physic, replied the Marchioness, has almost divested itself of the prejudice of observing certain seasons of the moon, as a proper time to apply its medicines; and perhaps natural philosophy has assumed it in her stead, that these superstitious notions may not be destroyed, but there may always be pretty near an equal dose of them in the world.

It must be confessed, however, answered I, that there may always be hoped some good effects from this diligent disposition, even though it be carried to such a degree as to become ridiculous: but we can never expect any good from negligence. You will see an evident proof of this, in that celebrated experiment of Sir Isaac Newton, before which all the antient idols of optics fall to the ground; those imaginary systems which supposed colour might be changed by refraction, reflection, the confinity to shadow; and in short that colour is nothing but a certain modification, as they express it, of light, which may easily be changed by these circumstances.

But Sir Isaac Newton has shewn the falshood of this opinion, and demonstrated that a ray, for example, red, well separated from all the rest, will constantly keep its colour in spite of any refraction or reflection it is made to suffer, or any other method that the fruitful invention of a naturalist can contrive to torment it. The same constancy will hold good in all the other colours, if they are well separated. The grand experiment which furnishes us with these agreeable and surprizing truths, is this which follows.

The image of the sun formed by the conjunction of a

prism and lens, is received upon a paper; by this conjunction the colours are much more unmixed and better separated than they would otherways be.

Having thus made a more perfect separation, the ray of different colours must pass successively through a hole in the paper, that they may be refracted by a second prism in order to prove whether this new refraction can produce any new colour. If it should, we must confess that colour is nothing more than a certain modification which the light acquires in passing through the prism; and then philosophers may set their imaginations to work, in order to find out what motions, figures, and the like, are necessary to produce this modification.

But on the other hand, if the ray constantly preserves its own colour without the least alteration, we must agree that refraction has no share in the production of colours, and abandon the antient system of modification: and all its ingenious delusive dreams will vanish at the rising morn of the Newtonian truth.

Now the experiment we are upon, demonstrates that a homogeneal ray, red, yellow, blue, or of any other primary colour, is not in the least altered, by a new refraction, nor even by a great number of refractions which it is successively made to suffer. It is not changed either in its colour or degree of refrangibility, which remains constantly the same. Thus, if two rays, one red, and the other violet, be made to fall one after another upon the second prism, with the same incidence, that is, if both the rays coming from the same point, fall likewise upon the same point of the prism: if the rays, I say, fall upon the second prism in this manner, the violet, after the second refraction, will strike the opposite wall in a situation higher

On LIGHT and COLOURS.

than the red, and the intermediate colours in intermediate situations, those which had suffered the greater refraction in the first prism, suffering the greater in the second likewise; all these colours will paint upon a white paper directly opposite to them, a little circle perfectly round, and not oblong like the image made by the first prism, and this circle will be of the same colour as the rays, without any addition or mixture.

I beseech you to stop and take breath, said the Marchioness; you were engaged in such a long period, that I began to think you would never come to the end of it. I should be sorry, Madam, answered I, if the length of the period has rendered me obscure, and made you loose so fine an experiment. No, no, said the Marchioness, I understand it very well. Does not all your meaning amount to this, that the homogeneal rays of light are immutable both with respect to colour, and degree of refrangibility? I am extremely rejoiced, said I, to find I may be as prolix in my periods as I please, without apprehension of obscurity, and may employ one as long as those of the Azolain dialoguists, to tell you that this is the experiment which Mr. Mariotte endeavoured to make, and by some misfortune found, that after the second refraction certain new colours were united to the red and blue. I know not how this happened, but probably it was from some defect in the prism which he employed.

The ill success of this experiment would have done the immutability of colour no small injury in the learned world beyond sea, if it had not been repeated in England before some learned Frenchmen, the motive of whose voyage was purely philosophical. This repetition of the experiment clearly demonstrated, that Mr. Mariotte, though otherwife an accurate obferver, has failed in fome of the circumftances neceffary to bring it to good effect. Thus were thefe two nations, more divided by their different ways of thinking, than by a little arm of the fea, reconciled upon this point.

This law of nature common to all nations acquainted with light, met with a lefs favourable reception in Italy, than in any other. The moft obftinate antagonifts of the Newtonian fyftem have rifen among us; there feems to be fome fatality in this, that a nation which the Italians once found fo difficult to fubdue by force, fhould in its turn find us the moft difficult to be fubdued by reafon.

In order to contribute my fhare to the eftablifhment of this law even among us, I caufed the fame experiment to be repeated at a place in Italy, celebrated for the learned men it has always produced, and neuter enough not to be fufpected of partiality. No minifter of ftate, faid the Marchionefs, could act more politicly in the choice of a proper place for the holding a congrefs. Within a very little, anfwered I, all my politics would have fignified nothing: for though we made ufe of Sir Ifaac Newton's own method in feparating the colours, and the chamber was extremely dark, yet a certain light of a blewifh caft always mixt itfelf with the colours refracted by the fecond prifm. It is true, this light was irregular and inconftant, but however, it was fufficient to ferve for an excufe to the incredulous.

This appearance give us a real inquietude: and we would never have flept in peace, if we had not, after much ftudy, found out the caufe. We obferved that the borders of the coloured image were not fo well terminated as they ought to have been, provided the prifm, by which it was coloured, had been good. We difcovered a light, round the edges, of the fame nature with that which was obferved to be mixed with the colours refracted the fecond time, and we perceived that feveral ftreaks of this light croffed the image from one end to the other. From all thefe circumftances it appeared, there muft be feveral irregularities in the prifm, as bubbles of air inclofed in the glafs, unevennefs in the furface, and other things of the like nature, which were probably the reafon why the light was irregularly refracted, and by this means rendered it impoffible for the colours upon the image to be perfectly feparated.

Various and repeated experiments made it evident that the fault of this apparent alteration of colours, which we obferved in the image, muft be imputed entirely to that irregular light which we had before fufpected to be the caufe, if we may call that an alteration which was nothing but the addition of one colour to another.

I congratulate you, interrupted the Marchionefs, that after fuch a difcovery nothing will hereafter difturb the tranquillity of your fleep. Heaven preferve me, anfwered I, from that cold tedious tranquillity, which is however the object of our defires. It is in philofophy as in all other human affairs, where the accomplifhment of one defire often gives birth to another.

When we had difcovered the caufe of this defect in our experiments, our next bufinefs was to find fome remedy for it. The difficulty of acquiring it was a new motive for our labour and inquietude.

Our prifms in Italy are of no other ufe than to amufe children, or hang up as a fine fhow in fome window in the country, and not for the fervice of philofophers, who are often too exact for artificers, and require a greater accuracy than is in the power of art to bestow.

We resolved to write to England, which has its Fawkeners for lapidaries, and its Grahams for clock-making, where, in short, every thing seems to be contrived for the service of the most curious and importunate naturalists, if fortune and our good genius had not unexpectedly furnished us with some which were just arrived from that country. These we esteemed as sacred, as the Romans did the article or shield which fell from heaven in the reign of Numa; and we could have wished for a Mamurius to make as many copies of these as he had formerly done of that.

With one of these prisms we renewed the experiment, and the coloured image, painted by it, emerged so beautiful, so well terminated, and so lively, that the other seemed no more, when compared to this, than a rough draught to a finished picture. The colours refracted by a second prism remained so immutable, that neither the most penetrating eye, nor even the *Zoilus* of the Newtonian system would have discovered the least alteration.

Perhaps, said the Marchioness, nature has reserved the merit of demonstrating truth to the English prisms, that is, to whose by those means she at first discovered herself. It would be a curious phænomenon, answered I, to observe such a partiality in nature, as for her to prefer such a prism made in London, to one produced in Murano. But the truth is, that if we consult her as we ought, she always answers the same, whether the prism be English or Italian, provided it be good and well worked; and the chamber, where the experiment is made, extremely dark.

if all these circumstances are rightly prepared, the colours, though refracted three or four times, will remain unchangeable, neither more nor lefs with regard either to colour or figure, than an object expofed to a homogeneal light, and viewed through a prifm. The variety of colours, the change of figure, and the confufion difcovered in objects looked upon in this manner, proceeds from nothing but their reflecting more or lefs all forts of rays, which, being afterwards differently refracted, produce all thefe irregularities.

If upon a circle of paper there fall at the fame time the red of one image and the blue of another, fo that the purple colour, compofed of both thefe, may appear, it will, when examined through a prifm, feem divided into two feparate circles, the one red and the other blue; and the reafon of this appearance is the different refraction of thefe two colours. If the yellow and green of two other images fhould fall at the fame time upon the paper, fo that it would be illuminated with four colours at once, it will appear oblong and divided by refraction into as many circles as there are colours, and thefe circles will feem placed upon one another. I know you are going to add, faid the Marchionefs, interrupting me, that if this paper be expofed to the light of the fun, who contains every fort of ray in himfelf, it will appear of a figure ftill more oblong, and painted with the colours of the rainbow; whereas, if it be illuminated by only one homogeneal light, it will alter neither its figure nor colour, when obferved through a prifm.

You muft forgive the weaknefs of human nature, Madam, anfwered I, if we generally finifh the fentence we have begun. It was referved for Sir Ifaac Newton and you, to understand nature by half a word, and find out natural philosophy, notwithstanding its uncertainty. It is superfluous to tell you that flies and other little objects placed in a homogeneal light, appear very distinctly to the eye with a prism; and the very smallest Elziver print may be read without any difficulty; but the same things will not have this effect, when placed in the heterogeneous light of the sun, because of the confusion and quantities of colours that arise.

In this case I abandon the prism to the disposal of poetry, to make use of it in comparisons, which do it no great honour. That celebrated author, whose fine ode you so much admired, compares it to false eloquence, which obscures the face of truth, lavishes its ornaments without distinction, and diffuses its glaring colour over every thing It is certain that the poet, in this comparison, means the prism which transmits the rays of every sort. And when it transmits only the homogeneal rays, said the Marchioness, may we not compare it to true eloquence and true spirit? For as it shews us the objects removed out of their place without any alteration, so true wit often surprizes us only by varying common subjects in a new manner.

You are so well acquainted with the prism, answered I that you may safely compare it with your own wit. But I know not what comparison you will find for the immutability of colours, unless you seek for it perhaps in your own heart; and then knowing that reflection has no more influence on that immutability than refraction has, you will be better acquainted with it than you at present are

If the colours with which bodies are variegated and painted were only a modification, which the rays of light acquire by being reflected from their various surfaces, a was once believed, a body which appears red in the light of the sun, would still remain red when placed in any other colour of the painted image, for instance, *blue*, because it could modify this blue colour refracted and modified already by the prism, as well as it does the light which comes directly from the sun.

But Sir Isaac Newton has proved by experiments, that every body placed in homogeneal rays is of the same colour as the rays themselves, without allowing, however, the supposition that bodies by reflection modify the light in such a manner, as to make it receive this or that particular colour. Thus all white, red, yellow, blue, green bodies, as paper, scarlet, gold, ultra-marine, and grass, in red rays appear totally red, in blue, totally blue, and so of the rest. The only difference consists in this, that all these various bodies, placed in the same homogeneal light, are not all equally luminous, but every body appears the most lively when placed in a light of its own colour, except paper, and all other white bodies which equally receive any colour, and may be regarded as the *Cameleon* and *Proteus* of optics.

Would this diamond then, interrupted the Marchioness, if placed in the rays of our coloured image, take indifferently any colour, and at one time be transformed to a ruby, at another to a topaz, an emerald or a saphire? So much the better, answered I, as it would dart only one unmixed colour, and all the varying splendors with which it sparkles in the direct light of the sun, would vanish in this homogeneal light.

It is very pleasant to observe how the fine dust or atoms in the air change colour as they pass from one ray to another, juſt as a river varies in its colour according to [the] various qualities of its bottom.

Other bodies, as I before mentioned, are not equa[lly] lively when placed in different coloured lights. The va[r]niſh, for inſtance, with which Martino, the emulator of [the] Chineſe art, makes ſo many fine curioſities, is extreme[ly] luminous in the red light, leſs in the green, and ſtill fain[t]er in the blue. On the contrary, the Lapis Lazzu[li] which has the honour to ſerve for a repoſitory to yo[ur] ſnuff, is extremely lively in the blue, leſs ſo in the gree[n,] ſtill fainter in the yellow, and almoſt dark in the red.

The ſame inequality holds good in bodies ſeen by a tra[nſ]mitted light, as is proved by glaſſes of different colour[s;] ſo that every body reflects or tranſmits, in great abundanc[e] thoſe rays which are of its own colour, and reflects o[r] tranſmits the other rays, in proportion as they are neare[r] or farther off its own colour in the order of refrangibi[li]lity.

It follows from hence, ſaid the Marchioneſs, that n[o] colour even that ſeems the moſt perfect, can be abſolutel[y] unmixed. And perhaps it will never be in the power o[f] art to dye a ſilk in ſuch a manner, as for it to reflect onl[y] one ſort of rays.

It would be more difficult, anſwered I, to ſort the va[]rious colours together, and flatter our ſight by the con[]cords of harmony, if they were all homogeneal and un[]mixt. In this caſe, all the delicacy of nature would be requiſite to find out the innumerable intermediate ſhades betwixt any two colours. But now as every colour is more or leſs blended with ſome other, we are by that means furniſhed with a more eaſy and expeditious way.

Hence it is that the gradation from one ſhade to ano-

r, though perhaps there may be several intermediate
es wanting, does not appear defective to our eye, which
covers in each the same basis of all the colours that sof-
is them, and serves for a support to the harmony.

There would arise other inconveniencies besides these,
coloured mediums did not transmit every sort of ray;
this would agravate a distemper bad enough in itself,
hich infects and tinges the whole body, and the eye it-
f with an unpleasing yellow.

Persons under such circumstances as these, when it is
ry improper to pay visits to ladies, would become abso-
tely blind, unless to yellow objects, and could see no
es but of those who are troubled with the same disorder.

A perfectly complaisant lover, replied the Marchioness,
his mistress should happen to be ill of this distemper,
ist clothe himself in yellow, a colour, which, though re-
rded with great veneration in China, is not looked upon
a good omen for lovers among us; and perhaps get the
indice in order to be seen by his charmer, and give her
proof of his affection.

So perfect a lover, answered I, would not be an improper
rson to prove this immutability of colours, if we had
more proofs to demonstrate it than what you have al-
ady seen. What remained to be shewn was, whether
e confines of shadow, with which the light is bounded,
e capable of making any alteration in the colours? This
ould have been fine sport for those naturalists who lay
old on every thing, in order to build a system.

Our philosopher put the colours to the test of this new
periment, and found nothing wanting in their constancy
hich maintains its ground, even when it happens that
ys of different colours cross and interfect each other; it

Q 2

appears, in short, to defy every thing judged capable
bringing any alteration upon them.

We must have recourse to romance, said the Marchi[oness]
ness, to find some equal to these colours, which do n[ot]
give place even to the *Ephesian Anthia*, a model of t[he]
firmest and most obstinate constancy, in spite of all tha[t a]
romancer can produce to make her at length ——— Wha[t]
answered I; resemble the matron her fellow-citizen, r[e]
plied the Marchioness. The constancy of these colou[rs]
must certainly appear very surprizing to ladies, answer[ed]
I. I do not doubt but the greater part of them wou[ld]
much sooner admit the system of Lucretius, who witho[ut]
so many experiments, affirmed not only that they are m[u]
table, but that any one colour may be changed into [all]
the rest.

DIALOGUE V.

Exposition of the Newtonian philosophy continued.

THE next morning, as soon as the Marchioness was up, she sent for me into her closet, not concealing that agreeable disorder which she knew her beauty could receive no injury from. I find indeed, said she, that your philosophy begins to grow a very serious thing. I can assure you, I have slept much less this night than before; I cannot tell whether this be the reason of it, but I find that philosophy and sound sleep do not agree very well together. My interrupted dreams have transported me into the region of optics, where I saw nothing but prisms, lenses, rays differently refracted, coloured images; in short, all those experiments, and all that philosophical apparatus which you described, arose successively in my imagination, like visions and fantomes. Whatever charms these things may have in themselves, I could never have imagined they would employ my thoughts so strongly at a time when it is not very customary to think of philosophy. No really, answered I, it was a time more proper to think on the philosopher. You are not to suppose, replied the Marchioness, but he had his share, and has no reason to complain of me. If this be the case, Madam, answered I, there is no great mischief done. I rather advise you to recal these dreams to your memory as often as you can, and you will be still the more sensible that they deserve it. How do you suppose it possible, continued she smiling, that I could think on these experiments without admiring the penetration and ingenuity of the philosopher who invented them.

a man who seemed directed by nature herself, in the method of tracing her laws? I perceive, said I, that you take the thing too seriously. In the present case I think you might be contented with the expositor. How! can be too serious? replied the Marchioness. We are examining whether colours be immutable or not, whether the rays of light be differently refrangible; we are building up and throwing down systems, and in short, our inquiries aim at nothing else than truth itself. Can you reasonably accuse me then of being too serious in matters of such importance? But these systems, answered I, and this truth however pompous they may sound to the ear, ought not however, to disturb our more agreeable dreams. It would really gain me a fine reputation in the world, if it were publickly known, that I had made you dream of lenses and prisms. We should act in things of this nature, as those, who study to make the best use of their passions, do with regard to love. These persons, who do not appear to be the most injudicious, never devote themselves so entirely to it, as to interrupt their more important concerns, but only as much as is sufficient to make them pass away two or three hours agreeably with that sex with whom it is hardly possibly to converse upon good terms, without at least a pretence of being in love.

You at once give me lessons in love and philosophy, replied the Marchioness. But you know when people first fall in love, they have little leisure for these grave reflections, but suffer themselves to be transported farther than they ought. This is exactly my case with regard to philosophy, in which I have hardly yet advanced one step. I am so little mistress of myself, that I have gone so far as to seek methods to confirm Sir Isaac Newton's system. After all you have told me, judge whether my tranfports were not very ftrong.

Let us fee, Madam, anfwered I, what they have produced, for we often owe the fineft things to ftrong paffions. The Iliad, Æneis, the poems of Dante and Milton, were produced in their moft vigorous time of life. To thefe may be added, at leaft for that veneration with which they are regarded by their countrymen, the Lufiade of Camoens, compofed in a time of the greateft revolutions and conquefts in Portugal, and the Araucana of the Spaniards, where the poet himfelf is the hero. Perhaps between the broken flumbers of laft night, your imagination produced fomething greater than all I have been mentioning.

I am afraid, anfwered the Marchionefs, that it will amount to very little. I was thinking, that if light is compofed of rays of different colours, which, blended together, produce *white*, we ought to examine whether thefe colours, after being feparated by the prifm, might not be mixt together again. I for a long time confidered, but with little fuccefs, in what manner this could be effected.

Sir Ifaac Newton himfelf, faid I, has delivered you from this trouble; for that method of confirming his fyftem which you mention is fo good, or rather fo evident and immediate a confequence of order, that he has made feveral experiments to that purpofe. I am now going to fhew you one of the moft celebrated, and at the fame time the moft fimple, to which this great philofopher was conducted by that fpirit of order which you poffefs in common with him.

The image of the fun made by a prifm in the dark chamber, is received upon a convex lens, that the coloured ray, which at going out of the prifm, diverged, may by the lens be made to converge and unite, and by this means be again blended together. I am quite aſhamed both of my ſtupidity and myſelf, interrupted the Marchioneſs. I had all the materials neceſſary for the execution of my idea, ready prepared to my hand; they only wanted puting together, and I had not the ſenſe to do it. You are greatly in the right, to be unwilling that a perſon ſhould hear the voice of philoſophy, who is incapable of making it an anſwer. I might rather, anſwered I, apply to you that famous ſaying of antiquity, *I wiſh with all theſe qualificatious, you were one of us.* You will find in optics themſelves, ſome conſolation for what you call your *ſtupidity.* Men, thoſe reaſonable and curious beings, lived above three hundred years before they found out that a convex and concave glaſs put together, would make a teleſcope; and though they had the materials every day at hand, were at leaſt indebted to mere chance for this uſeful inſtrument. It was a greater diſgrace to mankind not to diſcover it before, than honour to them that they found it at laſt. So that this uſeful and fine invention is of the number of thoſe which are ſtanding monuments of the weakneſs of human nature. You comfort me, replied the Marchioneſs, at the expence of mankind. ——But to return to our ſubject. I ſuppoſe that point beyond the lens, where the coloured rays are united, will appear totally white.

The rays, anſwered I, have no ſooner paſſed through the lens, but they begin to mix and efface each other; and they loſe the fine harmonious proportion eſtabliſhed betwixt them in the ſpaces of the coloured image, the original of the muſic of the eyes. When they are all confined at length, and incorporated together in the focus of the lens, they form a little circular image totally white, a republic, if I may use the expression, of colours, where they are all equally tempered together: The red can no longer display its lively flame, the green boasts no more the smiling livery of the spring, nor the blue the lucid robe of heaven, but all, blended together, restore the whiteness of the sun from whence they came, in such a manner, however, that as they recede from the focus, they again renew their splendor and colour, but in a contrary order, and the ravished eye again wanders from one pleasure to another.

You will easily understand how they came to be inverted, if you remember the two sticks crossed together, mentioned by Des Cartes, which you once believed to have a greater efficacy in explaining the phænomena of optics, than they really have. The appearance that the colours again make beyond the place where they were blended, demonstrates that the rays lose neither their colour nor quality, as some might perhaps believe, but that the whiteness, which happens in the focus of the lens, is produced only by their mixture

I now understand, said she, what you meant yesterday by saying, that the immutability of colours still remains, even when rays of a different colour intersect and cross each other; for if it were otherways, we should not see the prismatic colours re-appear beyond the place where the rays united.

This is the very experiment, answered I, upon which the immutability of colours was grounded; and all the experiments of Sir Isaac Newton have this peculiar and admirable quality, that each single one is not contented with demonstrating only one thing, as in the case of most others, but demonstrates many more at the same time. This arises from the close union, and almost geometrical connexion which the properties of light have between themselves.

Sir Isaac Newton's experiment, said the Marchioness, seems to resemble the battles of the antients, which often gained the victor a great number of provinces at a time. And those of most other philosophers, answered I, the battles of the moderns: the most noisy preparations, the most consummate contrivance, and the blood of millions, amount to no more than the taking a place, which perhaps might have surrendered in two months by treaty.

But to return to your experiment. I call it *your's*, because though you did not invent it, you saw the necessity there was for its invention, in order to complete the system. Our philosopher never quitted it till he had varied it a thousand ways.

It was necessary to prevent some one of the coloured rays from passing through the lens, in order to see whether the whiteness of the little circular image would by that means be changed.

This Sir Isaac Newton did, and intercepted the passage, sometimes of one colour and sometimes of another; and the whiteness ceased, and degenerated into that colour which arises from the composition of those colours which were not intercepted, but suffered to pass through the lens.

The want of any colour in the circular image, which is not suffered to pass, will be very agreeably discovered by looking through a prism, which resolves the image into its component colours, by giving them a different refraction.

If all the rays be transmitted through the lens, the

image will be white; but viewed through a prism, it will appear of all colours like the rainbow: if any ray be intercepted, this by the prism was discovered to be wanting in the image, till at last suffering only one colour to pass through the lens, this one colour too was seen by the prism.

If all the colours were successively intercepted by the teeth of a comb made to pass very swiftly over the lens, the circular image would remain white, and the different colours not be distinguished, by reason of the quick impression which they all successively make upon the eye.

You may perhaps have observed, that when a light torch is moved nimbly round in a circle, the whole circle which it forms in the air, appears on fire; and the reason of this is, because the sensation, which in the several places of that circle it raises in the eye, remains impressed till the torch returns again to the same place.

In the same manner, when the colours follow one another with an extreme rapidity, the impression of each of them remains in the eye, till a revolution of all the colours be completed. The impressions therefor of all the successive colours are at once in the same part of the eye, and jointly excite the sensation of whiteness there.

The same was afterwards proved by a wheel, whose circle, painted with the several colours of the prism, appeared white, when turned very rapidly round itself.

I must confess, said the Marchioness, that even if I could have found the experiment I sought for, I should never have been able to diversify it so many different ways, though the inconstancy which you, gentlemen, lay to our charge, might perhaps have given me no small assistance.

This inconstancy, answered I, which perhaps is not so

great a defect as some believe, was not wanting in S[ir]
Isaac Newton. With the most fertile, and almost poetic
imagination, he continually invented new experiment[s]
which, though different from each other, all concurred [to]
prove the same thing. They seemed to rise under h[is]
hands as the poets make flowers spring under the feet [of]
their beauties.

The coloured image, formed by the prism, becom[es]
white, when viewed through another prism, in such [a]
manner, that it contracts the image and mingles the c[o]
lours. I have observed the same phænomenon in the rai[n]
bow, which is the effect of a separation of the solar rays i[n]
the drops of rain opposite to the sun. It appears whit[e]
when viewed through a prism, turned in such a manne[r]
as to contract it and blend the colours together.

These who live near the cataracts of rivers, see a rai[n]
bow every day, when the sky is clear, formed by the s[un]
in the dashing of the water against the rocks; making peo[
ple have the opportunity of seeing this experiment muc[h]
oftener than we can.

I would, if possible, replied the Marchioness, have n[o]
thing to envy others. Though we have no cataracts, [a]
fountain will imitate the rain, present us with the colou[rs]
of the rainbow, and we may make our observations a[t]
pleasure. We will call this fountain, if you think prope[r]
The fountain of optics.

Till your garden furnishes you with proofs of the New
tonian system, answered I, as the gallery did with objecti
ons against the Cartesian, you may return to the dark room
there you will see that the whiteness of a paper placed ove[r]
against the coloured image of the sun, does not suffer an[y]
alteration, if it be placed in such a manner as to partak[e]

qually of all the colours; whereas, if it approaches nearer to one than another, its whiteness will be tinged with that colour which is next it. Is it possible now for truth to descend from heaven with a more shining train of proofs?

I was very confident, said the Marchioness, to venture my thoughts upon a thing, which cost Sir Isaac Newton so much study. How is it possible I could ever have found out the very least of these experiments, as easy and simple as they now appear? But in exchange, answered I, you can easily invent things that perhaps would have puzzled the philosopher. It is much more proper for you to know in what proportion to mix hope and fear, smiles and frowns, to prevent a lover's passion from growing languid, than to be exactly acquainted what quantity of different coloured powders is necessary to be mixed together to form a white. This is another experiment which our philosopher tried, that there might be nothing wanting to confirm his system. It is true, the white which arises from this composition, is dusky, grey, and obscure like the colour of ashes; and the reason is, because the colours of these powers are too imperfect and faint, compared with those of the prism, to make a lively clear white.

However if this mixture be exposed to the sun, in order to increase the force of the light, that dusky obscure white will become bright and clear, though it will never equal the strength of the paper exposed to the same light.

For this reason in coloured prints, one of the finest inventions of our time, which, with only three colours, perfectly imitate all the variety of painting, the paper is left uncovered for *strong clears* and *whites*.

Water thickened with soap, and agitated so as to raise a froth, is more proper to demonstrate that a composition of colours produces white. After the froth is a little ſettled, there will appear upon the ſurfaces of the bubbles which it is compoſed, different colours, which when viewed at a diſtance cannot be diſtinguiſhed from each other, the whole froth will appear perfectly white. This experiment has, beſide its being an agreeable one, this further advantage, that it is very eaſy to make.

Philoſophy, ſaid the Marchioneſs, from what I can diſcover of it, is like a game of cheſs, which upon any occaſion I ſhould make no ſcruple to call an ingenious pretext to waſte time. The very laſt piece in the one, or the leaſt experiment in the other, is often of the higheſt importance. A pawn, in the hand of a ſkilful player, may give check mate, and a little froth will furniſh Sir Iſaac Newton with a whole magazine of obſervations and diſcoveries. Half the world that preceded him had the ſame bubbles and froth before their eyes, without ſo much as ſeeing them. The antients themſelves would a thouſand times have obſerved and neglected them.

The eyes of the antients, anſwered I, were much better able to judge of the elegance of a ſtatue or a temple, than the importance of an experiment. Seneca was acquainted with a ſort of priſm, which, receiving the light of the ſun on one ſide, diſplayed to the eye the colours of the rainbow. All the explication which he gives of this phænomenon is, that there is really no colour, but only the appearance of a falſe colour like that on the neck of a dove, which appears and diſ-appears according to the motion of the eye and the change of its ſituation. This fine explication ſufficiently ſhews how very little the antients ſtudied nature and purſued her ſteps; for if Seneca had taken the leaſt trouble to examine his priſm, he muſt have ſeen the erence between the colours produced by that, and those [of] the neck of a dove.

A particular sort of microscope known to this philosopher, [and] which perhaps the antient artificers made use of in the [cur]ious ingraving of their intaglia's and cameo's, the e[nig]ma and admiration of our time, this microscope, I say, [com]posed of a ball of glass filled with water, had no bet[ter] fortune in his hands than the prism. He ascribed the [ma]gnifying of the objects viewed through this glass to a [qua]lity of the water, and not to the figure of the glass [wh]ich contained it.

The weight and other properties of air were known to [the] antients; and in order to explain how water ascends [in] a sucking pump, which is occasioned by this weight of [the] air, they had recourse to a certain imaginary horror [tha]t nature has for a vacuum: So that rather than leave [the] smallest space empty, she chose to violate her own laws [of g]ravity, and make the water ascend. And as one folly [pro]duces a thousand more, the great horror that nature [test]ified for a vacuum in this pump, extended only to a [cert]ain height, and beyond this perhaps was changed into [lov]e, for there she admits as great a vacuum in the pump [as y]ou could desire.

But to quote still more examples——Nero in his golden [pal]ace, one of the most magnificent effects of despotic power [in t]he universe, erected a temple of stone so very transpa[ren]t, that day-light entered into it even when the doors [wer]e shut. Pliny who gives us this relation, instead of [con]tenting himself with affirming that it was more transp[ar]ent than Alabaster, says, that it did not transmit the [ligh]t like other pellucid substances, but included it within

itself: if this had been the cafe, the temple muft have a[ppeared]
peared much more luminous by night than by day.

The antients were fonder of what raifed their admiratio[n]
than increafed their knowlege; and perhaps thought e[x]
periments, which are the only method by which we ca[n]
arrive to a true admiration of nature, were too immateri[al]
to imploy the attention of a philofopher, who ought to co[n]
fult nothing but reafon. They never imagined thefe e[x]
periments would one day lead induftrious pofterity to fuc[h]
an exactnefs as to fubject flame to the examination of [a]
balance, which was antiently regarded as a light fu[b]
ftance, for whofe fake they invented a particular fphe[re]
of fire where it was affirmed to afcend.

Nor could they forefce that thefe experiments could hel[p]
us to calculate how much we daily lofe by a continual i[n]
fenfible perfpiration, how many million tuns of water th[e]
Mediterranean fea perfpires in a fummer's day, how muc[h]
a man decreafes by the wearinefs of the mufcles from morn[n]
ing to night? In fhort, that they fhould inable us to coun[n]
terfeit nature herfelf; and by certain chymical mixture[s]
emulate her *Ætna's* and *Vefuvio's*, and imitate her thunde[r]
much better than their own rafh *Salmoneus*?

If an antient had been afked whether the phofphorus [of]
Bologna, for example, fhines by its own light, or by [a]
borrowed one, it is impoffible to know how many ridicu[-]
lous fancies they would have uttered by confulting reafon[,]
whereas a modern with a fingle experiment has put th[e]
matter out of all queftion. Pray, what is this *phofphorus*
faid the Marchionefs, this fubject of the abfurdities of th[e]
ancients and experiments of the moderns? It is a certai[n]
ftone, anfwered I, found in a mountain near Bologna[,]
which, calcined with fire, acquires the property of fhinin[g]

in the dark like a coal, if it has been exposed a little while to the light of the sun, or only to the open air. From this quality it has obtained the fine Greek name of *phosphorus*, which signifies a lucid body. This is an honour given almost to every thing appropriated to learned uses. An etymologist could not perhaps give a better name to this place than that of *phoslophus*, which in our language signifies the Lucid hill, and would thus consecrate it for ever to philosophy and learning. We are much obliged to your scholar, said she, for conferring so fine a name on this place which certainly deserves it.

The question, continued I, is at present reduced to this, whether the *phosphorus* only takes in and imbibes the light to which it is exposed, and from thence carried into the dark, shines with a borrowed light? or whether the external light puts its parts into such an agitation as to kindle a light which it contains within itself, which by this means loosed from its prison, if I may use that expression, emits itself from the phosphorus, which in this manner shines by its own light? This last supposition is more honourable for it, and better agrees with the fine name it bears.

In order to decide this point, a modern philosopher chose a sort of light which would shew whether the phosphorus, when exposed to it, inbibed any of its rays, and by that means reveal the theft of this new *Prometheus*. I already see, interrupted the Marchioness, how this modern proceeded. He placed the phosphorus in one of the colours of the prismatic image, in order to see whether it would acquire the colour as well as the light: if it did actually take the colour, it is evident that it imbibes the external light, and shines with a splendor not its own: but if it does not take the colour of the image, since colours are immutable and suffer no alteration, the light only agitates its parts, and as you express it, loses its splendor out of prison; and thus the phosphorus shines not by a borrowed lustre but its own, and ought rather to be compared with the sun himself, than Prometheus.

It is too true, answered I, that fine ladies can be just what they please. You would be extremely in the wrong if you hereafter complain of any want of sagacity in physics. What you have been describing is the very method which the Bolognese philosopher took; and by this experiment he confirmed to his fellow-citizen the phosphorus, the honour of shining by its own light. It is probable that the innumerable other phosphori of the same nature, lately discovered in France, owed their lustre to the same cause: these, by inriching philosophy with new wonders, have deprived the Bolognese of the honour of singularity, which it partook with only one other in the whole philosophical world. Do not diamonds, the most valuable phosphorus of nature, shine in the dark, because the external light kindles, and revives the internal light, of which they are a rich and inexhaustible treasure?

You may judge, replied the Marchioness, of my very great sagacity in philosophical affairs, when I never observed a phænomenon which I every day carry about me. Perhaps, Madam, answered I, you were never in a place dark enough to make this observation. Signore Baccari one day visited a lady in some indisposition, who was resting behind a screen far from the air, and in a place absolutely dark. The lady asked him whether he had not a light in his hand? which he denied; but she constantly insisting she saw something glitter, the doctor at last suspected it to be his ring which shone in that profound darkness, and perceived he had a long time, without knowing it, carried the phosphorus upon his finger. You may judge of the value he afterwards set upon this ring. He made innumerable experiments with it about the time that Mr. Du Fay, father of so many phosphori, found that diamonds had the same property. How empty and barren must the philosophy of the antients have been, said the Marchioness, and how copious, how charming is ours, whose observations enhance even the value of diamonds!

I will give you still greater evidence, answered I, how much the antients were to blame in their neglect of experiments, and you will be fully convinced that there is none even of those which seem of least importance, but what is of great service to natural philosophy. That froth we lately mentioned is an instance of this; for as little philosophical as it may seem to vulgar eyes, it was the principal thing by which Sir Isaac Newton found out the cause of those various and almost innumerable colours which we see in bodies.

He had discovered in general, that certain bodies appear of a certain colour, because they reflect one sort of rays more copiously than the rest, and other bodies of different colour, because they reflect a different sort; so that if light consisted of only one sort of rays, there could be only one colour in the world, nor would it be possible by refractions and reflections to produce a new one,

This discovery, which would perhaps have satisfied any other philosopher, served only to excite the curiosity of ours, and was but a prelude to innumerable others.

Why should this silk reflect the blue more freely than any other sort of rays? The reason is this.

If one of those bubbles which are formed by blowing

water a little thickened with soap, be covered with glass in order to prevent its being agitated by the air, it will appear tinged with a great variety of colours, which spread themselves like so many rings one within another, and incompass the top of the bubble. And in proportion as the bubble grows thinner by the continual subsiding of the water, these rings slowly dilate and overspread the whole, descending in order to the bottom of it, where they all afterwards successively vanish.

The variety of these colours depends on the unequal thickness of the bubble of water in different parts. But how to determine these inequalities is not so easy, and perhaps would have been impossible to any but Sir Isaac Newton, who examined these rings a thousand ways, guided by his constant tutor geometry, and a spirit of observation, whose fertility seemed to increase in proportion to the difficulties it encountered.

He discovered that a certain determinate thickness is necessary in a plate of water, for example, in order for it to reflect a particular colour, and a different thickness to make it reflect any other colour, and in general, that a less thickness is necessary to reflect the most refrangible rays, as violet and indigo, than those which are least refrangible, as red and orange; all this is to be considered with regard to the substance of equal density. But when the density in one substance is less than in another, as the density of air compared with that of water, a greater thickness will be necessary in the first than in the last, to reflect the same colour.

After the same manner he defined the thicknesses necessary for the transmission of colours. From the analogy or similitude between the plates of substances which he considered, and the particles of which bodies are composed, he demonstrated that their colours depend on nothing but the different thicknesses and density in their particles; whence it follows that some are more proper to reflect or transmit the rays of one colour, and others those of a different one.

This analogy holds good in many instances. Thus the one and the other are transparent: the leaves of gold and the particles of many other bodies transmit one colour and reflect another, just as the bubbles of water which we have been mentioning: these rings appear of a various colour when viewed in different situations; the same happens in certain silks, in the fine web of the industrious spider, and as Tasso sweetly sings,

> *The feathers so, that tender, soft and plain*
> *About the dove's smooth neck clofs couched been,*
> *Do in one colour never long remain,*
> *But change their hue 'gainst glimpse of Phœbus sheen.*
> *And now of rubies bright a vermeil chain,*
> *Now make a carknet rich of emeralds green,*
> *Now mingle both, now alter, turn, and change*
> *To thousand colours rich, pure, fair, and strange.*
> FAIRFAX'S Tasso.

This appears very evident in those powders that painters make use of; for when they are ground, that is, when their parts are subtilised, their colours change a little. Bodies may in some manner be regarded as stuffs, for their threads, every one in particular reflecting a particular sort of rays, the whole stuff appears of that colour which is the result of all the rays reflected from the several threads of which the stuff is composed.

But what becomes of those rays which are not reflected, said the Marchioness? Can you give an account of them? They are either transmitted, answered I, or stifled and extinguished, and are thus lost among the particles of bodies. A leaf of gold placed between light and the eye, is transparent, and appears of a greenish blue; but a collection of these leaves placed one upon another, loses both colour and transparency, the rays which pass through the first leaf being absolutely extinguished in passing successively through the rest.

White bodies, to continue our similitude, are stuffs composed of threads which reflect all colours; black, on the contrary, absorb and extinguish every sort of ray within themselves. For this reason, black bodies heat much more easily than any other; and a black cap, such as the English ladies wear in St. James's park, would not at all agree with your walks in the Italian sun.

White bodies, as they reflect and drive every sort of ray from them, heat with more difficulty than the others which imbibe and absorb the rays, and neither transmit or reflect them.

From the same cause arise the various colours which we discover in the air. The different density and thickness of the exhalations and vapours that rise from the sea and earth, paints the heaven with varying splendors, when rosy-fingered Aurora opens the portals of the morning, and calls back mortals to their several labours, or when Vesper invites them to an agreeable repose; it is difficult however, to trace a cause by which the colours at the rising and setting of the sun are almost all the same, and succeed each other in a certain order. But this we certainly know, that the several colours of different persons eyes proceeds from the difference of texture in the iris, which is that coat in the eye that incompasses the pupil.

The variety of fibres in the iris kindles in some the imperious look of a black eye, in others, the insidious sweetness of the blue. But it is not easy to assign a constant cause, why the northern nations should generally have white hair and blue or gray eyes, and we of a warmer imagination, not in a warmer climate, should have our eyes as black as our hair.

This system, however, will give us the explication of a phænomenon which is perhaps inexplicable in any other, and will thus make us a compensation for not being able to give a reason for every thing in particular.

The phænomenon is this: two transparent liquors, the one red and the other blue, cease to be transparent when we look through both at the same time. This phænomenon which so greatly surprised the person who first observed it, is only a consequence of the Newtonian doctrine. The one of these liquors transmits only red rays, and the other only blue. Hence it follows, that the rays, transmitted by the one, will be extinguished and absorbed by the other, and the eye which looks through each of them receive none. And this phænomenon is one of those whose explication becomes a demonstration of the system which is capable of explaining it.

That opinion, said the Marchioness, that blind people can distinguish colours by their feeling, now begins to appear credible to me: or rather, is it not another system? If our feeling was finer than it is at present, as fine as that of blind persons perhaps is, could not we discover the colour of a body by feeling the different thickness of its particles? And thus we should effect by our immediate sense,

what a Newtonian would by his calculations, if any one
should acquaint him with the hidden texture of bodies.

Your blind obfervers, anfwered I, might diftinguifh
colours by their feeling, even in the Cartefian fyftem
which you have now given up. For according to that
there muſt be a difference in the particles of bodies of different colours in order that the rays of light may be differently modified. A proof like this you perceive is too
ambiguous to deferve a place among thofe we have already
mentioned; and there is the fame defect in what is faid
of a fingular kind of barometer, which the Chinefe make
ufe of to form a judgment of the weather by. This barometer is a ftatue placed upon a mountain, which foretels the changes of the fky and air, by varying its own
colour.

But had we not better feek for a phænomenon nearer ourfelves in the nation of gallantry and politenefs
which can be explained by the Englifh fyftem alone? Why
fhould the belles of that happy country lay on more red
when they appear in the boxes at an opera, than when
they embellifh with their charms the agreeable walks of
the Thuilleries?

You lead Sir Ifaac Newton's fyftem, faid the Marchionefs, into places where you would have found it very difficult to lead its author. Not if you, Madam, anfwered I,
had been there.

The light of a candle is not fo white as that of the day;
it has a yellowifh caſt, and viewed through a prifm, yellow appears the moſt fhining colour in it. The lefs then
the Spanifh wool is charged, or in other words, the more
it reflects other rays befides the red, the ftronger will the
yellow appear, which is the predominant colour in this

rt of light; juſt as in a chamber where the light enters through coloured curtains, the objects in the chamber will the more eaſily take the colour of the curtains in proportion as their own colour is weak and faint. This is evidently a reaſon why the quality of Spaniſh wool ſhould be augmented for the opera, that neither the cheeks of the ladies, nor the eyes of their admirers, may loſe anything, but find the ſame advantages by the light of the evening as by that of the day.

In the Carteſian ſyſtem, this wiſe precaution would be entirely uſeleſs; for if the Spaniſh wool can modify the light of the day, it would in the ſame manner modify that of the evening, be it of what colour it will.

Muſt it not be a mortification, ſaid the Marchioneſs, for the ladies of this happy climate, if they ever have time to conſider it, not to have a ſyſtem in their own country able to explain this phænomenon in their vermilion, but be obliged to call a foreign one from beyond ſea to their aſſiſtance? So much the more glorious is it for this to extend its empire over all nations, even ſo far as to give them leſſons for the toilet. This is not the only one, anſwered

. If you would not have a blue appear green by candle-light, which might diſconcert the harmony of a ſuit of cloaths, and cauſe innumerable chagrins, you muſt be careful to chuſe it very clear, otherwiſe the blue rays mixed with the yellow, which the ſilk would reflect in greater quantities by candle-light, might perhaps make it appear green.

Theſe are the gordian knots of the optic ſcience, which his ſyſtem diſſolves without eluding the oracle. Theſe phænomena, inexplicable to every other ſyſtem, are without difficulty explained in this. Every ambiguous expli-

cation, every proof that has not the force of demonstration, is entirely rejected by the Newtonian philosophy.

An analogy, for instance, discovered between the production of colours and that of other things, which would
supply another system with a proof, can serve only for o-
nament and luxury to this.

It has been lately discovered, that insects, men, animals, and plants, instead of being continually re-produced
by nature, only unfold themselves from their respective
plants or seeds, in which they are really contained, whenever they find a proper disposition for it; that is, both
animals and plants wait for a proper repository, certain
juices, degrees of heat, and other things requisite to unfold them. In the like manner, colours are, not as
was once believed, produced at every refraction, or reflection, or some other similar cause, but unfold themselves,
if I may use the expression, from the bosom of light, which
contains them within itself, whenever it is refracted by a
prism, or reflected from the particles of bodies. And this
method of their production seems much more agreeable to
the universal laws and established order of nature.

After the same manner appears the colour of the rainbow, the coloured circles sometimes seen round the sun
and moon, and those of a certain light, which is often
seen towards the northern parts of heaven, and called Aurora Borealis.

Whatever riches and magnificence, replied the Marchioness, nature has displayed in so great a variety of colours,
she seems to have observed some frugality in their production. At least the Newtonian nature appears to me a better œconomist than the Cartesian. The first has made
light a magazine and reservoir of colours, which she pro-

...ced once for all, infusceptible of any alteration, only with
...certain difpofition that renders them capable of being
...parated from each other, and fhewing us by this fepa-
...tion a colour, which, all united and mixed together, they
...uld not do; whereas the Cartefian nature is every mo-
...ent obliged to give new rotations to her globules, and
...every refraction and every little circumftance, confider
...what manner to vary them. This muft be an infinite
...tigue to her, and a very great application of thought.

But thefe difpofitions, anfwered I, which the colours
...ve to feparate themfelves, and which you fo greatly
...dmire, however convenient they may be to nature by fpar-
...g her fo much trouble and thought, are fometimes very
...convenient to us.

Inconvenient! replied the Marchionefs. Is it not to
...efe we are indebted for the beautiful variety of the world?
...ow tirefome and unpleafant would it be for us to fee in all
...jects a repetition of the fame colour! You apprehend it,
...nfwered I, to be a great evil always to fee the world in
...iaro ofcuro, if I may ufe that expreffion, and to be oblig-
...to be dreffed always in the fame colour, and what is
...orfe, in a colour like that of your own complexion. You
...ay add, replied fhe, the dread of lofing a topic of dif-
...)urfe fo very pleafing to ladies.

All thefe misfortunes, anfwered I, and this terrible ad-
...tion of yours, would happen, if the rays had no difpofi-
...on to feparate from each other, or if they were all of the
...me colour. The Cameleon and wrinkled faces would be
...nfiderable lofers too. Some of thefe, without the trouble
...changing their fkin, are difcovered in the fpace of
...elve, or at moft twenty four hours to change their co-
...urs,

Astronomers, on the other hand, would gain no small advantage if the rays were inseparable and of the same colour. And what would not an astronomer sacrifice to determine the exact time of an eclipse of Jupiter's satellites, or to get a distinct sight of the ocultation of a star by the moon? These are a set of people whose looks are always directed to heaven, and have very little regard to our earth any farther than she is a planet, and upon that account enters into the celestial system. This is all they regard in her, and therefor would feel very little concern if the ladies of this planet were under an impossibility of changing every day the colour of their cloaths, or subject to many other the like inconveniences.

But what opposition, replied the Marchioness, can there be betwixt the separability of the coloured rays and the observations of these gentlemen, to make them quarrel with us for the pleasure we receive from this variety? There is a great opposition betwixt them, answered I, and you will be soon convinced of it, when I tell you that the separability of the rays is prejudicial to the perfection of telescopes, which astronomers regard as their very eyes. I before positively affirmed that convex-glasses, of which telescopes are composed, unite the rays, which, proceeding from a point, fall upon them into another point. But the truth is, I spoke rather with regard to what they should do than what they really do. You seem, said the Marchioness, to have represented these glasses in the same light as tragic writers do their heroes; for these generally chuse to feign them what they ought to be, rather than imitate their characters such as they really are.

It must be confessed, Madam, that I used a sort of poetic licence in telling you convex-glasses united the rays in to a point, for it is not so truly a point as a little circle. This circle, which is called the *abberration* of the light, proceeds from two causes, the figure commonly given to the lens, and that disposition which the rays of light have to separate themselves when they are refracted. But indeed the figure of the lens is but a very small obstacle when compared to that of the different refrangibility. All attempts therefor to render telescopes more perfect by giving a new figure to the lens, so as to make it unite the rays truly in a point, would be in vain.

In the golden age, of which the poets give us so many fine descriptions, when the rivers flowed with milk, and the oaks distilled the fragrant treasure of the bee, when the rams appeared in the meadows arrayed in native purple, and the lamb displayed its vived scarlet to the sun, before the hand of art had taught the fleeces to imitate different dies: in these happy times, it is probable, the telescope would have given a more distinct view of the objects of nature herself painted in their genuine and beauteous colours, when the heart of man, animated with purer passions, appeared without disguise, and love had not yet learned to sigh by custom or art, nor ever wept for any motive but joy. But in our iron age, in which both the passions and colours have degenerated from their original purity, whatever be the figure of the lens, the point where the blue or green rays unite, will always be different from that of the yellow and red; there must always be an abberration of the light; and that little circle will never become a point. This is a circumstance very inconvenient for astronomers, whose affairs require that every thing should be seen extremely distinct; but this circle where the rays unite instead of the point where they ought to unite, or the different refrangibility, which is the cause of their uniting thus irregularly, is a great obstacle to the obtaining the exactness which astronomers desire.

These accurate gentlemen, said she, must have patience, and pray for the return of the golden age. In the mean time they must limit their desires and wants as other reasonable men do, and be contented with the different refrangibility of the rays, instead of that very great distinctness in objects which they desire. It is not possible to have all things at one time in this world. Is the knowlege of so many fine and surprising properties of light so very small an acquirement, that they cannot be satisfied without something more? Their desires and their wants however are so reasonable, said I, and have so great a connexion with those of other people, that Sir Isaac Newton has thought upon a method of satisfying them. With his own hand he ground glasses for telescopes of a new figure, in order to correct the deficiency of ordinary lenses. Then was the time to have all, or hereafter hope for nothing.

While his mind was imployed in this thought, a new scene of optics opened to his view. He discovered the different refrangibility of the rays, laid aside the work he had begun, and invented a new telescope, in which a polished mirror supplies the place of what in ordinary telescopes is called the object glass, and which had the greatest share in the abberration of the light.

I myself have seen the first telescope of this sort, worked by those hands which had pointed to the planets their road in the vast desarts of a vacuum, and opened to geometry the immense career of infinity. This instrument is preserved in a city of England, where philosophy and politeness hold a mutual empire; with this are treasured up those prisms which the first time differently refracted the rays of light in the hands of our great philosopher, separated its emeralds, hiacinths and rubies, and unfolded to human eyes the celestial riches of the lucid robe of day.

In the reflection from a mirror, the rays are not separated as they are in being refracted through a lens, consequently the objects may be much more distinctly seen.

It has been tried in Italy, for even among us truth and Sir Isaac Newton have their admirers, that if a distant object, the one half red and the other blue, be viewed with an ordinary telescope, this instrument must be considerably shortened to give a distinct sight of the blue half, and on the contrary must be lengthened to shew the red distinctly; whereas in Sir Isaac Newton's telescope they appear equally distinct with the same length.

This reflecting telescope has besides another advantage over the ordinary ones; for one of Sir Isaac's invention, one foot long, is equivalent to one of twelve in the common sort; and one of forty foot to a hundred. And this is another convenience to astronomers who find great difficulty in managing long telescopes.

It is well for us, replied the Marchioness, that these astronomers will be now contented, for it seemed before a pretty difficult matter to please them. How is it possible, answered I, for them not to be satisfied with Sir Isaac Newton, who seems in every thing to have studied their advantage?

His system of optics, besides procuring them a more convenient and perfect telescope, has vindicated the honour of astronomy from an aspersion, which seemed in some measure to disgrace it in the eyes of the world. You are not ignorant that the honour of this science among men consists principally in its exact prediction of eclipses and events, no less observable to philosophical than to vulgar eyes. Thales of Miletus was reverenced among the Greeks like a god for having predicted the year in which an eclipse of the sun was to happen, that is, when the moon would be interposed betwixt us and the sun, and by that means deprive us of his light.

As astronomy successively became more perfect, what would have caused a temple to be erected to a Thales, would only disgrace a Halley, Cassini, or a Manfredi.

The observatory is required to shew the precise minute in which the eclipse will happen, and its exact quantity, or in other words, whether the moon will obscure the whole sun or only a part, and how much precisely the obscured part will be.

Not long since all the calculations of the most celebrated astronomers had predicted two total eclipses, whose principal merit consists in not being very common, and in introducing a sudden and unseasonable night. An event, which though foretold and expected, never fails to terrify that whimsical species of animals called men, that *asylum* of the strongest contradictions, nourished by long hopes, impetuous passions, the most evident truth and the most palpable error, capable of making attempts beyond the powers of his nature, and subject to fears which his reason contradicts.

All the philosophers got up very early on the days appointed for this spectacle, in order to prepare themselves for observation. They all waited in the midst of the eclipse to see the light of the sun entirely extinguished, and a most gloomy and profound night emerge from the splendor of a fine day. But the event was contrary to their

On LIGHT and COLOURS. 215

expectations. There remained round the moon a luminous ring which made some falsly take them for annular eclipses. When the sun is nearest to the earth, and the moon at the greatest possible distance, if there happens in these circumstances a central eclipse, as they call it, the moon cannot hide all the sun, but there remains all round its edge a luminous border resembling a ring. But astronomers gained nothing by this explication, which was of no signification in the present case, and the world was but ill satisfied with astronomy which is now believed an impostor. The one murmured and were discontented, while the other racked their brains to find the reason of this ring, which had the confidence to appear in spite of all their calculations.

Some laid the fault upon a luminous atmosphere which incompasses the sun, as our air does the earth, and became visible when the greater light was obscured; others accused the atmosphere of the moon, which, being illuminated at the time of the eclipse, appeared like a lucid ring. But unhappily for them the first was innocent, and the second seemed so doubtful, that it might appear rather a mark of their consternation, than an explication of the phænomenon.

I find myself greatly affected with concern, said the Marchioness, for these unfortunate astronomers, abandoned by heaven and earth, and in the utmost danger of losing their reputation. It is however the office of humanity to have compassion on the afflicted. They must have recourse, answered I, to the Newtonian oracles if they would silence the voice of calumny. These were the anchor of hope in the present calamitous state of affairs.

When the rays of light pass near the extremity of a body, they bend and incline towards the body itself, and are thrown into its shadow. If the edge of a knife be placed in a ray of light in a dark chamber, the rays, which pass at some distance from it, appear to bend and approach nearer its back. Grimaldo was the first who observed this quality, which is called the *diffraction* or *inflection* of light, and our philosopher afterwards illustrated it with many new experiments; and though he did not a great deal, desired to do still more.

The solar rays, which pass near the edges of the moon, must bend and cast themselves into the shadow of the moon herself. Observers then, who in the time of an eclipse are immersed in this shadow, must receive these rays bent from the edges of the moon, and see a luminous ring round her, a sort of twilight, resembling that which we see in the evening, and sometimes in the morning, at the horizon. The only difference between our twilight and this ring is, that the first is occasioned by the refraction which the light suffers in coming from the celestial spaces into our air, and the second by the *diffraction* which it undergoes in passing near the moon: but both are composed of rays which do not seem destined by nature for that purpose.

To give a stronger confirmation that this is the true reason of this ring, there have been made several globes of artificial moons, which exposed to the sun and full moon, have shown upon earth the effects of that diffraction which had appeared so fatal to astronomy in heaven.

Astronomers, replied the Marchioness, have certainly great reason to be satisfied with Sir Isaac Newton and his *diffraction*, which has delivered them from such eminent danger. But I must confess myself to be yet thoroughly discontented with it. Will you permit me to aſk, why thoſe rays, which paſs at ſome diſtance from bodies, muſt be inflected and bent? The idea which this new property of light preſents me with, is ſo very ſtrange that I cannot conceive it. I find, anſwered I, you are more difficult to ſatisfy than the aſtronomers themſelves. You deſire to know the cauſe of this *diffraction*. Well, I will inform you, but you muſt promiſe not to draw back and frown when I tell you it is the attraction which bodies exerciſe upon light. The attraction! ſaid the Marchioneſs, with an air of ſurprize. You ſay this either to laugh at my credulity, or puniſh my too preſumptuous curioſity. What! do bodies attract the light as a loadſtone does iron? What ill conſequences would ariſe ſuppoſing it were ſo, anſwered I? or rather how great an advantage has the ſcience of optics in particular gained from this attraction between light and bodies, as all natural philoſophy in general has from the univerſal attraction of matter, of which that between bodies and light is a conſequence?

Attraction is the key of all philoſophy, the great ſpring that actuates the frame of nature; the univerſal and myſterious force diſcovered and calculated by Sir Iſaac Newton, propoſed to the examination of philoſophers by the great lord Bacon, and obſcurely ſung by the Britiſh Homer.

The Marchioneſs recollected herſelf, and looked very attentively in my face to ſee whether I ſpoke in earneſt. Do you tell me ſeriouſly, ſhe replied, that all bodies are attracted? This is quite a new world to me where I am an utter ſtranger and foreigner. Do not be diſcouraged, ſaid I, for this has happened to many profeſſed philoſophers who have exclaimed againſt this attraction, affirming, that to admit it is introducing into philoſophy certain occult qualities which the antients supposed in bodies, such as simpathy, antipathy and the like, whose number multiplied with the phænomena themselves, by the assistance of which, they in an instant explained, or rather perplexed every thing.

They farther add, that it is recalling those occult qualities from those colleges of Europe, where ignorance still affords them asylum, to introduce them into true philosophy, from whence they for the happiness of mankind had been banished by the authority of reason.

But all these objections signify nothing, for attraction is so far from being an *occult*, that it is an extremely evident quality of matter, on which clearly depends the explication of *diffraction*, refraction itself and innumerable other things. It is not a name without reality, invented to explain two or three appearances, but a general principle diffused through all nature, and extends from the smallest grain of sand to the greatest planet. The Peripatetics resembled those antients, who for every little river or tree, nay even for the fever or the cholic, created a new deity. But Sir Isaac Newton, when he affirms, that light in passing near the extremity of bodies is attracted by them, does not pretend by that to give a complete explication of *diffraction;* all he undertakes is only to point out that property of matter on which the explication of *diffraction* depends, but the cause of this property is to seek. This he commits to those philosophers who have superfluous time enough to throw away in search of a thing which appears above the reach of human faculties. In short all that Sir Isaac Newton attempts is to establish facts, and the general properties of matter, and from these geometrically to deduce phænomena and effects; and this is th order we have hitherto observed in our discourse upon light and colours.

This new property, replied the Marchioness, is of a nature which my thoughts cannot so easily come into. This is one of those historical facts of which it is impossible to get a perfect intelligence without entering into the cabinet. I understand, or think I understand, how the rays of light are differently refrangible. This, among many other things, is very intelligible. But that bodies should attract the light, and that at a certain distance too, and in general that every thing should be mutually attracted, seems to me very difficult to conceive.

Some remains of Cartesianism, answered I, which you are not yet entirely free from, deceives you in this point. Perhaps you have hitherto flattered yourself that refraction arises from some one of those causes which in treating upon the Cartesian system were rendered so familiar to you, and upon this account you think refraction more intelligible than *diffraction*. Sir Isaac Newton himself appears in some places to have indulged the prejudices of this sect. In order to speak the language then current in philosophy, he said, that attraction perhaps might be the impulse of a subtile matter proceeding from bodies. But in fact, after he had proved the heavens to be empty, and the celestial bodies mutually attracted in those vast spaces, what room did there remain for the impulse and subtile matter? He seems to resemble certain authors, who, to make their history agreeable to any particular nation, are sometimes obliged to intersperse it with fabulous episodes, and give it the air of a romance. Is it not a great reproach upon mankind, that even the truths of Sir Isaac Newton were

T

obliged to use some little artifice in order to meet with reception among them?

Is not this rather an artifice of yours, interrupted the Marchioness, to surprize me by a motive of honour, and in this manner make me believe that I have no better conception of the subtile matter than of attractions, or how bodies should be endowed with motion, for example, than with that which you rightly term a *mysterious* force?

Your illusion, answered I, proceeds from hence, that you are familiarized to one idea and not to the other. You every day see bodies move and mutually communicate their motion, but you have never seen them attract each other. You are surprized at attraction, while motion appears to have no difficulty. In this you differ from philosophers who, like poets, for the solution of any difficult point are obliged to have recourse to the divinity for the explication both of motion and its communication.

A Portuguese accustomed to reverence spectacles upon the nose of the gravest persons, as a mark of the gravest dignity, would probably be surprized to see a Chinese mandarin let his nails grow to an enormous length for the very same reason. And the cause of his being surprized in one case and not in the other is, that a long habit has connected in his mind the two ideas of honour and spectacles which have nothing in common with each other; but has not connected those of honour and long nails. I shall at least deserve more compassion than the Portuguese, replied the Marchioness, because the surprize of seeing matter united to attraction instead of motion will, I believe, be common to all countries.

As universal and excusable as this surprize may be, I answered, it must however at last submit to reason. If you had never seen bodies move, it would have been impossible for you to guess how motion would be joined with extension and mutual impenetrability, which would be all the qualities you would then have been acquainted with. It is observation which has made you admit this property in matter, and observation must make you allow attraction. We are as yet but children in this vast universe, and are very far from having a complete idea of matter; we are utterly unable to pronounce what properties are agreeable to it, and what are not. We see bodies in very near the same manner as a person who should receive his senses by little and little. It would certainly be great temerity in him to affirm that there cannot be a property in matter capable of moving the eye, and should assign as a reason for this assertion, that he had never been able to observe any such property.

This person would not act like the Cartesians who form a world and a man just as their own caprice directed them; he would grow more cautious in limiting the power of nature and pronouncing the qualities of bodies, in proportion as he should acquire new senses, which would every day furnish him with fresh discoveries of these things.

Philosophers may be said in some degree to acquire new senses, or rather those they before had become every day more refined, and are by that means in a capacity of perceiving what perhaps they had once no idea of. Hence it evidently follows, how very cautiously they ought to proceed in assigning the number of properties in matter. It signifies nothing to say that some are more intelligible than others, for to speak ingenuously, they are all equally mysterious to us.

Will you any longer make a difficulty, Madam, to admit attraction as a property of matter when it is proved so many ways, and principally by the heavenly phænomena, which give the most shining testimony to a thing that you yourself so evidently demonstrate the truth of? I assure you for my part I shall never look for any farther demonstration of it than what you afford.

But I, replied the Marchioness, shall not be so easily satisfied, for I have need of the daily attestation of all heaven itself to convince me of a thing which yet appears so strange and surprising. It is absolutely needful then, continued I, to give you a full conviction of it. And indeed it would be doing a great injury both to Sir Isaac Newton and yourself, to endeavour to make you believe a thing without giving you good reasons. I am sorry this system cannot be explained to you with all the force of those demonstrations and calculations which accompany it; without these you must certainly lose a great deal. I will have patience, said she, if I cannot see it in all that lustre in which it would appear to a mathematician, and will act like those virtuosi, who, when they cannot get a picture, content themselves with the copy of it. I flatter myself, you will render it as like the original as possible. It is at present too late, I replied, for this expedition. To-morrow we will ascend into heaven, and from thence bring attraction down in triumph to earth. Some astronomical facts and propositions in geometry, which you may safely believe upon the word of Sir Isaac Newton, shall serve for a hippogryph, or flying car, to transport us to the skies.

DIALOGUE VI.

Expofition of the NEWTONIAN *univerfal principle of Attraction, and application of this principle to Optics.*

CONCLUSION.

THE next morning, the Marchionefs no lefs impatient for attraction than fhe had been for all the reft, after a few fhort compliments, began. It is now time to mount our hippogryph, and give him the reins. He will not grow weary, anfwered I, for a little journey, if I can remember certain horrible numbers.

All the planets revolve at various diftances round the fun, who is almoft nine hundred thoufand times bigger than the earth, and forms a centre of their motion, while he remains in the tranquillity of a majeftic repofe. Neareft the fun, at a diftance however of thirty two millions of Englifh miles, is the little world of Mercury; then follows the lucid orb of Venus fifty nine millions diftant; then our Earth eighty one; Mars, at one hundred and twenty three; the enormous bulk of Jupiter four hundred and twenty four; and the vaft and flow-moving Saturn, feven hundred and feventy feven millions of miles.

Thefe all preferve this natural order in their motions, that thofe neareft the fun complete their revolution or orbit in a fhorter time, and the moft diftant in a longer: thus Mercury finifhes his revolution in eighty eight days, Venus in two hundred and twenty four and fome hours, the Earth, as you already know, in a year, Mars in about two years, Jupiter in almoſt twelve, and Saturn in about twenty nine years and a half.

There is ſo great a dependance and relation between the periodical revolutions of the planets and their diſtances from the ſun, that if we know the diſtances of any two, of the Earth and Jupiter for inſtance, and the periodical time of one, ſuppoſe of the earth, by a certain rule we may find the periodical time of the other.

I ſhould have a much clearer idea of your meaning, ſaid the Marchioneſs, if I had firſt read Foutenelle's plurality of worlds to convince me of the motion and agility of the earth. As you are now ſo great a proficient in philoſophy, I replied, you muſt ſeek the true demonſtration of this motion in England.

There have been obſerved certain appearances in the ſtars which ſome imagined to be conſequences of this motion; but others who examined them more ſtrictly, have diſcovered theſe appearances to be contrary to the laws of ſuch a motion. The motion of light which is a conſiderable time in coming from the ſtars to us muſt ſtrangely vary their appearances, and ought to be conſidered in conjunction with the earth's motion round the ſun, in order to give a right deciſion of the queſtion.

The ſagacity of the Engliſh philoſophers has in fact united theſe two motions, and by this means they explain theſe ſurpriſing and various appearances which in any other ſyſtem are abſolutely inexplicable. And thus we have attained to the certainty of a thing proved a thouſand ways, but never ſtrictly demonſtrated by any.

The five planets, in whoſe number we may ſafely replace our earth, are called *primary*, to diſtinguiſh them from other subaltern planets which revolve round a primary, as the moon does round our earth, the four satellites of Jupiter round that planet, and five round Saturn; and these subalterns are called *secondaries*. These last agree with their primaries in observing this order, that the nearest complete their orbit in a less, and the most distant in a greater time; and they keep this law with the same exactness and the same relation as their primaries do.

Another law in which the primary and secondary planets agree is, that they do not describe equal parts of orbits in equal times, but such parts of orbits as to make their areas equal. That you may better understand this other law of their motion, you are to suppose that the orbit of a primary planet is very near a circle which the sun is not placed directly in the centre of, but a little on one side. Imagine a line to be drawn from that point of the orbit where the planet now is, to the sun, and another line to be drawn from that point where the planet will be twenty four hours hence. The space contained betwixt the two lines drawn to the sun, and that part of the orbit which the planet has described in twenty four hours, is called the area, and will be equal to such another area that the planet will describe in twenty four hours more; and thus in equal times the areas will be always equal.

The areas then, as astronomers express it, are *proportional to the times*. Thus, if instead of twenty four hours we put twelve, which is one half, an area described in those twelve hours will be only one half of the area described in the 24; and so, if we take a third or fourth part, will be the third or fourth of those described in the first time; and if that time be doubled, the area described in it will be doubled likewise, and so on. This law which the primary planets obferve with regard to the fun, the fecondary planets obferve with regard to the primary, round which they revolve; and this primary is the fame to its fatellites as the fun is to the planets of the firft order.

I am extremely pleafed, faid the Marchionefs, with the agreement between thefe two forts of planets. I regard the fun as monarch of the immenfe planetary realm, in which the primary planets are the grandees and nobles; fome of thefe poffefs certain diftricts where they exercife the fame jurifdiction in little which their fovereign does in great, but all fhew their dependance by revolving round him alone.

Our Earth is in poffeffion of a little province, where fhe exacts obedience from the moon; and though fhe cannot vie with Jupiter or Saturn who have a great number of dependants, fhe is certainly fuperior to Mars, Mercury and Venus, who have none.

Your fimilitude, anfwered I, would be jufter in the Cartefian fyftem of vortices where thefe jurifdidictions feem very well eftablifhed; and it would be the more fo, becaufe, this philofophical poetry is fond of imbellifhing itfelf with comparifons and fimiles, and fometimes makes them even ferve for reafons. But the two laws I have mentioned to you, will not fuffer it. Indeed it is pity we are obliged to abandon thefe vortices, that prefent the mind with fo clear, fo natural and fimple an idea. The planets, fay the Cartefians, revolve round the fun, becaufe a certain fluid in which they are immerfed turns round too, and carries them with it like little fkiffs forced along by the current of a river. The fecondary planets revolve round their primaries for the fame reafon.

Nothing feems to be more evident than this. But the

misfortune is that these planets are not contented with
barely turning round, but will do it by certain inviolable
laws that entirely destroy all these imaginary systems.

Either these two laws cannot agree with the vortices,
or agree so ill, notwithstanding all the efforts to that purpose, that one of their most illustrious defenders confesses,
after all he has done in their support, he doubted whether
those who refuse to admit them would not be confirmed
in their opinion by the very manner in which he has endeavoured to defeat it. Besides these vortices are pressed
by so many other insuperable difficulties, that heaven itself
seems to have conspired in the destruction of this fine
poem.

Far be it from us, replied the Marchioness, to oppose
the decrees of heaven. On the other hand, I cannot reconcile myself to the idea of a poem in philosophy. What
is this philosophical poetry to which I cannot assign a place
in my thoughts? It ought to content itself with influencing the passions of men, but it has nothing to do with the
single passion of philosophers, which is truth.

The Newtonian principles, answered I, have inspired
you with very rigid sentiments. But this poetry, that
thinks itself too much limited in the vast field of human
passions, shall give you no farther trouble. Comets, the
most declared enemies in all heaven to their vortices, will
I believe be sufficient to overthrow it, for they seem to be
made expresly for the destruction of systems.

It has been established, by virtue of I know not what,
but however the philosophers have very readily believed,
that the matter of the heavens was incorruptible, and that
every thing flourished in a perpetual youth, insusceptible
of the changes and vicissitudes which happen here below.

The comets appear at laſt almoſt naked, but in their approach to the ſun are clothed with a formidable tail, of which they gradually diveſt themſelves as they recide from him, and ſo return back naked as they came. And in this manner is the ſyſtem of the incorruptibility of the heavenly regions, in great danger of being overthrown by theſe impertinent comets. And this perhaps is the reaſon why they were degraded from their celeſtial ſeat as worthleſs meteors formed by the vapours and exhalations of our lower world. But they would not remain long there; for beſides many ancient philoſophers who conſidered them not as one of the tranſient, but durable works of nature, the aſtronomers who muſt have their ſhare in a thing above us, aſſure us, that they are very diſtant from the earth, and ſome of them farther off than the ſun himſelf. Theſe comets, ſaid the Marchioneſs, are very bad omens to ſyſtems, if not to crowned heads. Theſe were not all the troubles, ſaid I, which they gave philoſophers. When they were placed among the celeſtial bodies, they could not agree with that ſolidity which had been granted to the heavens upon the word of Ariſtotle; in order therefor to abide their demoliſhing and breaking to pieces the whole univerſe in their paſſage through theſe Ariſtotelian heavens, it was neceſſary to reſolve upon making theſe laſt fluid.

When the heavens were thus made fluid, they became vortices, againſt which theſe factious comets renewed their enmity with more violence than ever, to deſtroy an agreeable imagination received by the world with ſo much applauſe, and which was defective in nothing but truth.

Some comets have made no difficulty to croſs the orbits of all the planets, proceeding almoſt directly from the ſuperior part of the vortex to the ſun; others have moved in a courſe abſolutely contrary to that of the planets, without meeting, either in the firſt or ſecond caſe, any reſiſtance in their motion, which muſt neceſſarily have happened, if there was a certain matter that whirled round the ſun, and this at ſeveral diſtances from him with the ſame rapidity as the planets ſuppoſed to ſwim in thoſe vortices. Their motion would have been ſo weakened, that turning round the ſame way as the planets do, they would ſoon have yielded to the irreſiſtible force of the vortices, not unlike the unfortunate barks, which, guided by an unſkilful pilot or a malignant ſtar, are ſhip-wrecked in the horrible cataracts of the Chineſe rivers, notwithſtanding all the ſtruggling they can make to the contrary.

In ſhort, theſe comets have in every inſtance acted directly oppoſite to the laws of vortices. So that to reſcue them from the continual injuries they receive from theſe implacable enemies which lay hold on every occaſion to commit all ſort of hoſtility and impertinence, I ſee no other remedy than to deſtroy and baniſh theſe unhappy fluids for ever from the ſyſtem of the world.

Your expedient, replied the Marchioneſs, is no leſs violent than that ſometimes uſed in war, when one party deſtroy and ruin a country which they cannot defend againſt the enemy. And thus they make the ſame ſacrifice to their weakneſs as you do to truth. This is a ſacrifice at which I cannot be diſpleaſed, eſpecially as it puts me into a better capacity of liſtening with more tranquillity to the new principle upon which the celeſtial ſyſtem is built.

Sir Iſaac Newton, continued I, founded his ſcheme in geometry, which we may call his native country. He began with demonſtrating, that if a body in motion is attracted towards a point either moveable or immoveable, it

will describe about this point equal areas in equal times
and in general, that the areas will be proportional to th[e]
times; and on the contrary, if a body describes round [a]
moveable or immoveable point areas proportional to th[e]
times, it will be attracted towards that point, that is, th[e]
body will have such a tendency towards the point, that i[f]
every other motion which impells it a different way shoul[d]
cease, the body would directly unite itself to that point
just as bodies here below, when left to themselves, fal[l]
directly upon the earth.

This principle, interrupted the Marchioness, is equall[y]
applicable both to the primary and secundary planets
Each of these describe areas proportional to the times
round the point about which they turn, if the sun, our
earth, and Jupiter, may be termed points. The primary
planets then are attracted by the sun, and the secundary
by their respective primaries about which they revolve.
Is not this a necessary consequence? It is without dispute
absolutely necessary, answered I. But remember, Madam,
this is a deduction of your own. The punishment is just,
since you have made so much difficulty to admit the principle of attraction.

You say then that there is a force in the sun which attracts the planets to him, and after the same manner, a
force in the planets that attracts the satellities; and this attractive force joined with another by which they all move
from west to east, is the reason why the first revolve round
the sun, and the others round their primaries, in a certain
order.

The antients, in order to explain this difficult phænomena, built solid heavens, and created intelligences to put
them in motion; on the other hand, Des Cartes had em-

On LIGHT and COLOURS.

[em]barrassed the whole universe with the great and magnificent apparatus of his vortices. But after all, the motion of the heavenly bodies is by Sir Isaac Newton reduced to the most simple yet the most noble phænomenon in the world, which has been rendered much more familiar in Europe, than is agreeable to some persons. In short it is no more than that of a bullet, which would of itself proceed in a direct line, if the attractive force of the earth did not oblige it to move in a curve. The bullet very soon falls to the earth, because the greatest force we can possibly give it, is but little when compared to the vast extent of this globe. If it were possible for human weakness to throw one from hence beyond Peru, it is demonstrated that we should acquire a new satellite; it would like the moon revolve about our earth, only its motion being necessarily very soon weakened from the continual resistance of the air, while the gravitating force would lose nothing of its strength, this new moon would at last fall and destroy every thing it lighted on, after we had heard it make a horrible hissing over our heads.

All this you explain in two sentences; an evident proof of the significancy of a lady's words. What you have said is certainly a great deal, but not all. It still remains to know by what law this attractive force acts, that is, whether it be the same at all distances from the sun, or whether it grows weaker in proportion as the distance is greater. I will resolve you this question, the Marchioness replied, when you have furnished me with as many hints for that purpose as you did when I told you that the planets are attracted by the sun; and I hope you will afterwards make as genteel a commentary upon me as you did in the other case.

U

That law, anſwered I, of deſcribing areas proportion: to the times obſerved by every particular planet, furniſhe Sir Iſaac Newton with means to diſcover the attractiv force of the ſun; and that other law which they obſerv of deſcribing their orbits in a greater time in proportion they are at a greater diſtance from the ſun, and that wit a certain relation between theſe times and their diſtance helped him to find out that the attractive force diminiſhe as the diſtance from the ſun increaſes.

The attractive force diminiſhes with this proportion that it is always ſo much leſs as the ſquare of the numbe which expreſſes the diſtance from the ſun is greater. I order to underſtand this cyphering, which perhaps at fir ſight may appear very formidable, it is neceſſary to ac quaint you that the ſquare of any number is nothing bu that ſame number multiplied by itſelf; as four for inſtanc is the ſquare of two, becauſe twice two makes four; tha is, two multiplied by itſelf gives four.

I may now ſafely venture to propoſe you a problem that as you have lately explained the phænomena of natura philoſophy, you may now undertake the ſolution of ma thematical problems: after this I do not ſee what you ca do better than to ſhew ſome ſort of gratitude, and diſcove the truth to him who has conducted you into its moſt ab ſtruſe and retired paths.

The problem I ſhall propoſe to you is this: ſuppoſe th earth's diſtance from the ſun to be one, and Jupiter's di ſtance from him to be about five, conſidered with reſpec to that of the earth, the queſtion is to know how muc the ſun's attractive force will be diminiſhed at the diſtanc of Jupiter?

Give me a little time to conſider, anſwered ſhe, wit

On LIGHT and COLOURS. 233

...me impatience, for the folution of a problem is no trifling affair. You have informed me that the attractive force is fo much lefs, as the fquare of that number which expreffes the diftance is greater. The fquare of one which is the earth's diftance from the fun, is one. And at the diftance one, anfwered I, the force is fuppofed to be one, and the queftion you are to refolve is, how much that force will be diminifhed at the diftance of Jupiter from the fun, which is five. The fquare of five, anfwered fhe, with great quicknefs, is twenty five. If the attractive force muft be fo much lefs as this fquare is greater, it follows that in Jupiter it is twenty five times lefs than in the earth. Is not this the folution of your problem? and may not I, like Archimedes, run crying about, *I have found it, I have found it?*

Yes certainly, anfwered I, but not in the fame circumftance as he did, when his impatience was fo great as to make him run precipitately out of the bath. The mathematicians ought rather to act as Pythagoras did upon the difcovery of a certain truth, and facrifice a hecatomb to folemnize this day which gives them liberty to embellifh and brighten their gloomy catalogue by your name.

The law that the attractive force obferves of growing weaker at various diftances from the fun, is the very fame to which all other qualities that flow from bodies, are fubject; as fmell, found, heat, and which moft nearly concerns us, light. Thus when you believe yourfelf to have folved only one problem, you have in reality folved two. Is then, replied fhe, the light of the fun as well as his attraction twenty five times lefs in Jupiter than with us? The very fame number, anfwered I, ferves equally for both. After the fame manner you will find that the attraction,

U 2

the light and heat of the fun, muft be ninety times lefs in Saturn than with us. The twilight of our fartheft Laplanders would be there the fineft fummer days, and in the moft raging dog ftar of that planet, our feas hardened with perpetual ice, inftead of fwift failing veffels, would groan under the weight of heavy chariots; whereas in Mercury, they would even in the depth of winter be diffipated into thin vapors, occafioned by this extreme proximity to the fun, and would thus leave their bottom dry, and prefent to pilots a horrid gulph, a dreadful view of the terrors of the deep; and to naturalifts a beautiful fcene that would furnifh them materials to enrich their mufæums.

You fee, anfwered fhe fmiling, how many fine difcoveries I have made without perceiving any thing of it. It is however true, that great affairs are generally brought to pafs we know not how, and we are at laft amazed to find them effected.

In human affairs, anfwered I, it is afcribed to their good fortune, if the Cæfars and Alexanders, after propofing only one end, acquire another which they never dreamed on. It often happens, that thofe very perfons who are called fortunate, gain that name by fome events very different from what they intended. The inventor of gunpowder, it is probable, propofed a quite different end to his ftudies than the difcovery of a fecret to deftroy mankind with the greater facility; and that perfon who found a new world fought nothing but a more expeditious way to the richeft part of the old.

On the other hand, in true natural philofophy and geometry, the Cæfars and Alexanders are more common. It is very feldom that we find only what we fought. The discovery of one truth frequently produces many others which appear in spite, as it were, of those who seemed to disregard them. Any one who carefully seeks that law by which the attractive force ought to act at various distances, will at the same time discover that universal law by which all the qualities which flow from bodies are governed. Natural philosophy afterwards illustrates this general truth with peculiar experiments, and in some measure translates the obstruse hieroglyphics of the learned tongue into vulgar language. That decrease of the attractive force which immediately concerns light, is demonstrated by a very easy experiment, which we may try this evening, if you are not already sufficiently tired with philosophy and experiments.

Suppose one single candle to be placed in a room, and recede from it at such a distance as not to be able to distinguish the characters of a book, or a letter, unless perhaps it were a billetdoux, which may be read at any distance.

Place yourself afterwards at a distance twice as far from the candle as you were at first. In this situation the force of the light must be, according to the established law, four times less than it was at the first distance. The letter then cannot be read with the same distinctness as it was at first, unless the light be *quadrupled:* that is, the law requires that in the proportion as the light grows weaker, the square of the distance must increase. And this proves the experiment to be true; for the letter at the second distance is then only read with the same distinctness as at the first, when three more candles are added to the single one, or, in other words, when the light is *quadrupled.*

Considering how very easy people are apt to forget

these objects in their abfence which made the greateft impreffions upon their mind when prefent, I cannot help thinking, faid the Marchionefs, that this proportion in the fquares of the diftances of places, or rather of times, is obferved even in love. Thus after eight days abfence, love becomes fixty four times lefs than it was the firft day, and according to this proportion it muft foon be entirely obliterated: I fancy there will be found, efpecially in the prefent age, very few experiments to the contrary. I believe, faid I, that both fexes are included in this theorem, which feems rather to follow the cubes of the times, which is certainly more convenient, and requires only four days for an intire oblivion. But, in genneral, I believe we may without fcruple eftablifh the proportion of the fquares, for eight days are common enough to cure the moft vehement paffion. You alone have power to reverfe this theorem, and make the rememberance of you, and with that a defire of feeing you, inftead of diminifhing, increafe according to the fquares, or rather the cubes of the times. No! no! faid the Marchionefs, gallantry muft never deftroy a theorem. I am willing to enter into the general rule, and fhall think myfelf exceedingly happy if I have been able to eftablifh any thing fixed and conftant, in an affair fo inconfiftent and wavering as love. If geometry, anfwered I, was permitted to get fome footing there, it would in a little time produce wonders. The conclufions would be the moft ready and elegant imaginable.

But to be ferious, faid fhe: our conclufion in natural philofophy was, that the attractive force of the fun diminifhes in proportion as the fquares of the diftances increafe. I fuppofe the attractive force of the planets will follow the fame proportion with regard to their fatellites. The fatellites, anfwered I, which turn about any planet, obferve the fame relation between the diftances and the times of their revolutions, as the planets themfelves do that turn about the fun. This is evident in Jupiter and Saturn, who have more than one fatellite, and confequently the law of their attractive force will be the fame as that of the fun.

In the earth, who has only a fingle fatellite to her fhare, this is not altogether fo evident. But what reafon is there why it fhould not be the fame in one as in the other?

If we had another fatellite revolving about our earth at a diftance different from that of the moon, it would difcover whether the attractive force of the earth obferves the fame law as that of the fun, Jupiter and Saturn. This defect however is fupplied by the bodies which we fee every day fall upon the furface of the earth; for we are to believe that the force which would make the moon fall if fhe loft her motion from weft to eaft, is the very fame that makes bodies here below fall upon the furface of the earth when they are left to themfelves: for fince it is demonftrated that the earth has an attractive force, it is evident we muft in this force feek the caufe of gravity, another phænomenon, which the vortices have been as unfuccefsful in the explication of, as in that of the planetary motions.

If we could raife bodies from the earth to very confiderable diftances, compared with that at which we ftand from the centre which is very great, we fhould fee the force of gravity prodigioufly diminifhed in them. A man of war of a hundred guns, for whofe formation a whole foreft was cut down, and a whole mine exhaufted, would be overfet by the flighteft breeze of a zephyr. The famous *ftone-henge* upon Salifbury plain, the fruitful source of fables both to the learned and ignorant, those Colossian heaps which are held together by the force of gravity, would be no more than houses built of card. The velocity in the fall of heavy bodies would be considerably retarded. Bombs, those artificial thunders, would not be more terrible than so many flakes of snow. But these experiments are impracticable; one of the greatest distances we can attain is *Pike Teneriff*, which is only about three miles perpendicularly high. Besides the air would be too thin for respiration, and the cold, which must be exceedingly sharp at a greater height, would render any experiment fatal to the philosopher who had the courage to undertake it.

Nature, replied the Marchioness, has in this case denied us the means of being complete Newtonians. She has here confined us within the bounds of probability. If the attractive force observes a certain law in the sun, Jupiter and Saturn, why should not the same force observe it here on our earth? In this point, answered I, we have no reason to complain; we have no need of higher mountains, and a different constitution of air, in the present case. All these things, and the defect of another moon, are, as I before observed, supplied by the bodies which fall upon the surface of the earth. We may compare these bodies to the moon herself; and thus instead of probability we shall have evidence, and be even in this point good Newtonians.

It has been deduced from observation, that if the moon should lose her motion, and fall towards the earth, that force which would set her a falling would be three thousand six hundred times less than the force which makes bodies fall upon the surface of the earth. You see how well this agrees with our principle. The moon is distant from the centre of the earth, where the attractive force chiefly resides, sixty times as far as these bodies: the square of sixty is 3600: the attraction then of the earth to the moon is diminished in the same proportion as the square of the distance is increased; and this is exactly agreeable to the established law in Jupiter, Saturn, and the Sun.

If the moon should happen to fall upon the earth, replied the Marchioness, it would present a fine and agreeable sight to the Newtonians: they would certainly have neither curiosity, eyes, nor calculations for any thing else. This might very easily happen, answered I, if every thing was body, as the Cartesians affirm; and those antient Gauls, who were apprehensive the heavens might one day or other fall upon their heads, would have some reason to fear it in the system of their own Des Cartes: for it has been demonstrated that if this planet was to move in a place absolutely filled with matter, without the least empty space, let this matter be supposed ever so subtile, fluid and æthereal, her motion from west to east would be so retarded that it would soon grow weaker, and at length totally fail. And thus yielding to the force of gravity, she would fall precipitately from heaven to earth, and we should no more behold her that triform goddess we before admired, but a stranger banished from the most shining of her three kingdoms, and no longer the ornament of heaven amidst the friendly silence of the night.

The other planets would undergo the same fate if they moved in a plenum. These would all, some sooner and others latter, fall into the sun, and supply that immense volcano with a greater quantity of matter. He would then reign the sovereign of a depopulated empire: his animating light would shine in vain: Not a single planet would be left to partake his pleasing influence, nor receive from him the seasons and the day; for both the comets and we with our moon should be stifled in him, if we met with an obstacle in our æthereal road. This would be a new punishment to an age fruitful of crimes, in the system of that English writer * who makes the glorious body of the sun the mansion of grief, and the seat of eternal despair.

I assure you, for my part, I should be one of the first, continued I, who would run to see the moon fall upon the earth. What an agreeable spectacle would it be to see, in proportion as she approached to us, that face, that mouth and nose, which we discover in her rather by our imagination than our eyes, gradually transformed into great mountains, vallies, plains and the like, which must certainly fill the vulgar with great astonishment: nay even philosophers themselves, who can never sufficiently master those two great enemies of reason, fancy and prejudice, could not help looking on this phænomenon, without some degree of surprise. As she approached still nearer, said the Marchioness, should not we descry the sighs of lovers, dedications to princes, courtiers promises, vials filled with the judgment of our sages, and all the other lost things which Ariosto places there? You have not read the Plurality of worlds, answered I, and therefor are not capable of seing the greatest curiosities in that planet; since you are not yet acquainted with the force of a *why not*, which peoples the whole universe.

But one thing which I should take great pleasure in observing, if the moon should really happen to fall, is,

* Mr. Swinden in his treatise *of the nature and place of hell.*

what treatment the earth would give the moon in going to receive her.

What! replied the Marchioness; is it a point of ceremony established among the planets, that if a satellite should fall upon its primary, the latter must go meet it, and shorten its way? This ceremony, answered I, is founded upon mutual and reciprocal attraction. If the earth attracts the moon, why should not the moon attract the earth? The attraction which the earth exercises upon the moon, is lodged in that matter of which the earth is composed; why then should not the matter of which the moon is composed exercise its attractive force upon the earth, since all matter is entirely the same, and only differently modified in different bodies? Besides *action*, as the philosophers express it, *is always equal to reaction*. You cannot press this table with your finger, but it will be equally re-pressed by the table. Thus if two little gondolas made of cork, in one of which is placed a loadstone, and in the other a piece of iron, are set a floating upon the water near each other, the loadstone will run as fast towards the iron as the iron does towards the loadstone; and if either of them be hindered, that left at liberty will spring towards the other, which could not happen unless the iron attracted the loadstone as much as the loadstone itself does the iron, or, in short unless the attraction were reciprocal.

I perceive, said the Marchioness, what will be the conclusion of all this. The sun attracts the planets, and consequently the planets attract the sun: the secondaries attract each other, and are all attracted by the sun, and all attract him. Does not this multiplicity, this chaos of attractions, perplex not only me but the system itself too? No,

Madam, anfwered I, it happens in this juft as in the new geometry, of which I was fpeaking to you the other day, in which all thefe innumerable orders of infinitely fmall quantities, inftead of perplexing, render it more fubtile and perfect.

This mutual attraction, diffufed through the univerfe and all its parts, retains the wandering planets in their orbits, and connects all bodies, the earth, and us ourfelves, by ftrong though invifible ties, and regulates and tempers every motion in fuch a manner, that its exiftence and irrefiftible laws are every inftant apparent.

In thinking on this reciprocal attraction, faid the Marchionefs, fomething comes into my mind, which I dare not however propofe as an objection to a fyftem which the philofophers themfelves cannot venture to oppofe. It appears to me that if there really was fuch mutual attraction, we muft fee the effects of it in thofe bodies which furround us, if not every inftant, at leaft very often, juft as we difcover from their gravity the effects of that general attraction which the earth exercifes upon them.

When any little, light, body, as a feather for inftance, is placed near a palace, a hill, or any thing whofe attraction is very ftrong, why do not we fee it prefently obey the force which attracts it, and move, as it fhould do, towards the palace or hill? When our mind is poffeffed by a very ftrong paffion, anfwered I, what is the reafon we do not feel the weaker, unlefs it be that the ftrong paffion attracts the whole foul, fo as not to fuffer the weaker to make any impreffion upon it, and thus we become infenfible to all the reft which are not in themfelves either light or weak.

The furious paffion of Phædra for Hippolytus in Racine,

does not permit her to feel that strongest passion in the fair sex, the desire of beauty. Her ornaments and her whole dress are in that disorder which perhaps neither the absence nor death of her Theseus could ever have produced in them.

I comprehend you, replied the Marchioness, notwithstanding your parabolical method of explaining this point. The very great attraction which bodies feel from the earth, if I may use that expression, renders them insensible to that of the other bodies which surround them. Bodies, answered I, attract only in proportion to the quantity of matter they contain. I make no scruple of using mathematical terms to you, for to use any other would be an affront to a person who has given the solution of a problem.

Thus a ball of gold, besides many other advantages, has a greater attractive power than that of wood, because it has a greater weight; and if the first be a hundred times heavier than the last, that is, if it contains a hundred times greater quantity of matter, it will have its attractive power a hundred times stronger.

Now the attraction of this great ball upon which we stand is diffused on all sides, and draws every thing to it with an immense force, and by that means hinders us from perceiving the effects of that particular force, which the little balls by which we are surrounded exercise upon each other.

A globe of the same density with the earth, and of a foot diameter, attracts any little body placed near its superficies, twenty million times less than the earth does. The attraction of the highest mountains, as that of Pike Teneriff, Ararat, or even the Apennine, notwithstanding

X

the pompous defcription made of it, is abfolutely imperceptible.

But it is not fo with the effects of the lunar attraction upon this vaft collection of waters that fome philofopher made the firft principle of things, which by the eafy method of navigation joins the moft diftant countries, and tranfports to us from another world thofe balms and aromatics which feafon the European entertainments. You feem, replied the Marchionefs, to have a very lively fenfe of our obligations to the ocean, and the advantages we receive from it. But has not the philofopher amidft thefe entertainments forgot the attraction of the moon? The ocean, anfwered I, every day fhews us the effects of this attraction, which extend its empire throughout all nature. The ebbing and flowing of the fea, a phænomenon, which in the moft polifhed age of Greece, Alexander the Great took as a mark of the divine difpleafure, and with which the Romans in the golden age of Julius Cæfar were but very little acquainted, is only a confequence of that attraction the moon exercifes upon the fluid and yielding part of our globe. Chapelle in his celebrated voyage, that model of polite and agreeable wit, believed that no one but a watergod could penetrate into its caufe.

This god relates to him, that when Neptune was made governor of the fea, the rivers went to congratulate him. The Garonne upon this occafion retained fomething of the haughty temper of his country, and his compliments were not fo fubmiffive as was neceffary in addreffing that power who raifes the tempeft by a fingle nod, and with an *I will*—— filences them to a profound calm.

The punifhment which this arrogant river received for his crime, was to be repelled twice a day back to his fource.

all the rivers which flow twice a day into the ocean undergo the same fate. But why, answered the Marchioness, should the other rivers who were not guilty of this afcon behaviour suffer the same punishment as the Garonne? If it was permitted to make objections to superior powers, I would humbly propose this to Chapelle's Neptune.

You may make objections equally strong, answered I, to all the human systems that have been made to explain this phænomenon. Some affirmed the respiration of this vast animal the earth and the sea to be the reason of it; others a great gulph in the northern ocean near Norway, which emits a vast quantity of water and afterwards swallows it up again, a most fatal circumstance both for the fishes and philosophy which have the misfortune to be plunged in its deeps. The ancient Chinese, who supposed their little country of four leagues extent, to be the universe itself, asserted that two great nations, descended from a certain princess, the one inhabiting the mountains, and the other the sea-shore, had frequent wars with each other, and this was the reason of the flux and reflux according as either of the combatants was drove back towards the mountains or the sea.

Such perhaps was the infancy of philosophy among all, even the most sagacious people. The explication of Des Cartes which was produced in a later age of the world is ingenious enough to render it agreeable, but not accurate enough to be true. The same English philosopher who cast an impenetrable obscurity over vision, by involving it in his contractile and expansive forces, has endeavoured to involve this phænomenon also in the same unintelligible terms. This gloomy fancy diffused itself like an universal contagion over the whole face of things, and infected the whole fyftem of natural philofophy.

According to this opinion, the moft fimple and evident method of explaining the tides, is by afcribing their caufe to the contractive forces of the earth and moon, by which the one raifes and the other depreffes the water. To thefe he unites the expanfive force of the fun, which, though always contrary to the contractive, yet upon this occafion muft act in concert with that of the moon. Thefe unintelligible terms, which have not fo much as the fafhion to fupport them, can imply nothing in the author but a vehement and vain defire of giving his name to a new fyftem of errors. Thefe philofophers, faid fhe, appear to me the priefts of Chapelle's divinity: their explications at once difcover both the temerity and weaknefs of their philofophy. Our's, anfwered I. takes delight in difficulties, and comes off in triumph; amidft the thorns we are fure at leaft to meet with rofes.

That portion of the water immediately under the moon and neareft to her, muft be more ftrongly attracted than the reft which fhe looks obliquely on, and which is at the greateft diftance from her. The ocean then muft flow together from all parts, and be heaped into a mountain of waters whofe fummit will be under the moon herfelf.

The earth itfelf is a little attracted by the moon, but that part of the water which is directly oppofite to the part under the moon is leaft attracted, becaufe it is at the greateft diftance.

This part then will be as it were forfaken by the earth which a little follows the attraction of the moon, and will there form the fummit of another watery mountain, and thus there will be two, the one totally oppofite to the other.

The ocean then muft fwell, and in fome meafure lengthen itfelf in that part where the moon is, and in the part oppofite to her, and thus from the figure of an apple be changed to that of a lemon, whofe extremities will always follow the moon in her diurnal courfe; fo that the water will be at one time depreffed, and at another raifed, both in the fame place.

In every part of the ocean there will be two tides, during the time which the moon employs in returning to the fame point of the heavens. When fhe is at the meridian, the waters muft be raifed, and when fhe fets, depreffed; another elevation when fhe is at the meridian of the Antipodes, and another depreffion when fhe rifes.

All this muft unavoidably happen if the whole earth was covered with deep waters, and they immediately obeyed the attractive force of the moon. But becaufe there is fome time neceffary for the accumulating the waters, and their courfe is interrupted by fhores, ftraights, iflands, and the like, there are fome irregularities in the tides.

Thefe irregularities however are not fo great, but twice in every twenty five hours, which is nearly the time that the moon employs in her return to the meridian, we fee the veffels laden with the riches of the univerfe go up with the tide along the filver waves of the Thames, and twice defcend with the reflux to go in queft of new treafures. And this advantage, which in the fyftem of Chapelle was inflicted as a punifhment, all the rivers which flow into the ocean enjoy.

Have our Mediterranean rivers, faid the Marchionefs, ever offended the moon, that they are not fuffered to enjoy the same advantage? Perhaps they have affronted her as the Garonne did Neptune.

The ſtraight, anſwered I, by which the Mediterranean has a communication with the ocean, is too narrow for ſo great a ſea, and is diſadvantageouſly ſituated, ſince it looks towards the weſt, to receive the great flood of the ocean that follows the moon from eaſt to weſt.

On the other hand, the tide which is formed in the Mediterranean itſelf is too much interrupted with iſlands, ſhores and ſtraights, for the flux and reflux to be very conſiderable. In the Adriatic, on the contrary, it is more ſenſible than in any other place, becauſe the ſea is very narrow, juſt as the motion of a river is moſt apparent and ſeems moſt rapid when confined between the arches of a bridge. In our fine city founded by the gods upon the ocean, the viciſſitudes of the flux and reflux carry the fluctuating gondolas from one ſide to another, while the gondolier ſits at his eaſe, and ſinging to the agreeable light of the moon, teaches the ſea nymphs the flight of Erminia, or Rinaldo's love.

The changes of the tides are ſtill leſs perceptible in the Baltic ſea, the Mediterranean of the north; for this ſea bordering upon the frozen regions of the Pole, and very diſtant from the courſe of the moon, ſeems more adapted to ice and rocks than to warmth and attraction.

In the ſhores of the ſouthern and oriental oceans, to Japan and China, the tide is very conſiderable by reaſon of the extent of the ſeas; and in our ocean its effects are incredibly prodigious. There are coaſts near Dunkirk, where the ſea draws back for the ſpace of ſeveral miles, and afterwards on a ſudden returns and overflows the ſame ſpace again, alternately covering and diſcloſing thoſe ſands ſo

On LIGHT and COLOURS. 249

very fuspicious to failors, not without sometimes disturbing the ladies in that country, who venture to walk upon the margin of the sea, whose very shores are faithless and deceitful. These are a sort of natural sea fights, where at some parts in the day two armies may engage on dry land, and at others, two fleets, at least such as those of the ancients were.

In some rivers the tide rises to more than fifty foot high, especially if the sun and moon act in conjunction to render the flood considerable.

Though the moon may be regarded as the empress of the ocean, the sun however has his share in it. Notwithstanding he is at a greater distance from the earth than the moon is, yet in return he is so much greater, that it is not proper he should remain idle, but lend his part to the production of the tides. The rest of the heavenly bodies have no sensible influence in this case, the vast distance they are separated from us renders them too small.

When the moon is in her quadratures, the tides are less than at any other times in the month. The reason of this is, because the attractive forces of the sun and moon crossing each other, are as contrary as is possible to the swelling of the sea in the same situation.

On the other hand, when the moon is new or full, she is in the same direct line with the sun in respect to the earth, their forces are united, and then the tides are highest.

It is to be observed however, that the motion begun in the waters, and retained for some time within them, must be some days after the new or full moon, before it produces the greatest raising of the sea. So in summer, the heat of mid-day that remains in the air, being added to the following heat, less intense in itself, is the reason why we have not so great need of the assistance of the fan to supply us with fresh air at noon itself, as we have some hours after.

The greatest of all the tides happens at the new or full moon of the equinoxes; for besides the conjunction of the solar and lunar force, the waters in this case acquire a greater agitation; but because the sun, notwithstanding our freezing, is nearer to the earth in winter than in summer, these great tides do not happen at the precise time of the equinoxes, but a little before the vernal, and something later than the autumnal, that is, in the month of February and October.

In Mercury, Venus, and Mars, the tides are governed by the sun alone, though they must be almost insensible in Mars, because that planet is at so great a distance from him. In Jupiter and Saturn, the distance from the sun is so very great, that he can have absolutely no influence over the tides. They will confound each other according to the caprice of the satellites, the great number of which will render them very irregular.

If we knew the time of Saturn's rotation as we do that of Jupiter's, and were as well acquainted with the geography of both, and the quantity of matter contained in their moons, as we are with their distances and revolutions, we might conjecture the quantity and period of their tides, and send tables of them to their pilots. Thus are we again transported by attraction into heaven, to vast and remote worlds, where this powerful quality holds its most conspicuous and shining seat.

By the help of this, replied the Marchioness, we can travel thousands of miles in an instant, and are well recompensed by innumerable great and shining truths. A French author, I answered, a zealous propagator of this system, like us transported by attraction to these distant worlds, thinks with great probability, that the moons of Jupiter and Saturn as well as ours had once been comets, which passing near enough to these planets, to remain confined within the sphere of their attraction, were constrained to revolve round them, and thus degraded from the rank of primary to that of secondary planets.

Saturn has obtained so advantageous a situation as to make him the most happy in the number of his conquests. For the same reason he was able to acquire a fine ring, that incompasses his body, and which was formerly the tail of a comet that unhappily passed too near him.

This Saturn, replied the Marchioness, must be very terrible to the comets that approach a little too close to him. He must be the same to them, as the *Cabo tormentoso*, to which avarice afterwards gave the name of Good Hope, was to the Portuguese. It must, I fancy, have been a very agreeable sight to see Saturn at once adorn and enrich himself with a splended ring, while the poor comet was forced to pursue its journey, spoiled of the honour of its shining train.

He robbed it of nothing, answered I, but what it enjoyed at another's expence, according to the supposition of a certain French author, who assures us, that the comet, in crossing the atmosphere of the sun, had from thence stolen its tail. But the Newtonian opinion is, that the tails of comets are formed and composed of certain vapours arising from the comets themselves, when they are near the sun.

Is it not a very great advantage, replied the Marchioness, to be possessed of a system that supplies even the imagination with the most pleasing amusement, by those

strange and surprising events which it renders possible?
And all this, answered I, only by the force that among us
makes a stone fall to the earth. This attraction, said she,
appears to be the same in the hand of nature, as the subject of a composition in that of a skilful musician. Be it
never so simple, yet when he undertakes it, he will diversify it a thousand ways, and make it appear every moment
new; in short, he will find enough in it to form the most
harmonious concert in the world.

Nature, continued I, wants no other subject at once to
regulate and vary those innumerable and vast planetary
systems, which probably revolve round the fixed stars, those
luminous and attractive suns that chear the night, and
which we debase by giving them the names of our miserable heroes. But why should these heroes, said the Marchioness, remain unmoved and fixt? If they have a mutual attraction, how comes it to pass, that they do not
approach each other and run all together? You have, perhaps, some other parable ready which only waited till I
should propose a difficulty. No, Madam, answered I, unless you take it for a parable when I tell you that this would
exactly happen, if the number of those suns was not infinite. Those which are upon the superficies of this immense sphere of suns would be united to those next them,
because they would not have any thing to attract them
a contrary way, and by that means keep them in their orbits. And thus these successively running into those next
them, and these last into others, they would be all heaped
together. By this means in a little time there would be
in the whole universe only one sun of an enormous size.

But what is the number of these suns? What are the
limits of their sphere? Is not the centre of it throughout,

and the circumference in no place? The difficulty you have moved would be alone sufficient to induce us to multiply the stars, *ad infinitum*, even if we had not a thousand reasons besides.

I am quite lost, replied the Marchioness, in this infinity of suns, and planetary worlds; pray let us return to our own. We are possessed of a system capable of diversifying it to infinity, if we were so fond of infinity as to desire it. And a system, answered I, which predicts and gives a reason for the very smallest irregularities that can happen. After attraction and its laws were established, how sublime a geometry was requisite to find out what path the planets must keep in the spaces of heaven, and how much more sublime still to foresee exactly how much they would deviate from that path in the constitution of the present system? The vastness of the objects renders general rules difficult, and the niceness of the variations renders the exceptions still more difficult.

The sun who was esteemed immoveable in the centre of the system, and imagined himself exempt from any irregularity, is found however to be subject to it; for the attraction between bodies is always mutual, and every cause must have a currespondent effect proportioned to its activity. As the planets and sun reciprocally attract each other, he must be sensible of their force; so that to speak with the utmost rigour, he continually changes *his*, as they vary *their* situation with respect to him. After all our speculations then, replied the Marchioness, to prove the immoveability of the sun, we are at last reduced to make him move again. Had it not been better, continued she, with a certain malicious smile, to adhere to the common opinion without giving ourselves all this trouble?

Do not you act like those persons, who after employing their reason to divest themselves of popular prejudices, are afterwards obliged to have recourse to the same reason to resume them, if they have an inclination to live and converse with their fellow mortals?

Our case, answered I, is extremely different. The question then was to make the sun revolve about the earth with such a motion, as to run a million and a half of miles in one day. But at present the Earth herself continues to revolve about the sun, and he has no other employment than to approach or recede a little sometimes towards one and sometimes towards another side of the common center of the whole system. This motion is insensible in astronomy, and is in fact only a mathematical subtlety with which I thought myself obliged to make you acquainted. If the planets were all on one side, you are sensible that their united forces must act upon him with the greatest possible strength, in order to draw him back to themselves and make him recede from the center of the system: they would not however attract him, considering the enormity of his bulk, any more than one of his diameters. I am very willingly convinced of my error, said she. The sun, who, notwithstanding his vast size, is subject to the general force of gravity, may serve for an example to great kings, whom neither the extent of their fortune, nor the superiority of their station, can ever exempt from an observation of the universal laws of humanity.

Our moon, continued I, is at present subjected by attraction to the minutest and most exact calculations of astronomers. Her very irregularities, her caprices are reduced to certain and constant rules. Comets, those enemies to systems, who made still greater resistence to the power of numbers than the moon herself, are at length obliged to revolve about the sun. And though their orbits are much more oblong than those of the planets, yet they observe exactly the same laws.

By observations made upon their appearances, philosophers have assigned what orbits the comets must run in this system, and these in fact are the orbits which they really have run, almost with the same exactness as the other planets. Notwithstanding the imperfect observations left us by the ancients concerning comets, the moderns have ventured to predict the return of some of them, in the same manner as they do eclipses. And indeed, what is there which this system might not authorise? A Titian could easily judge of a picture from a rough draught.

The prophecy of that ancient is now fully accomplished, who even in his time foresaw that posterity would calculate the periods and predict the returns of these bodies, these eternal monuments of the ignorance and weakness of human nature.

It is expected that the comet which appeared in 1658, will return twenty three years hence, and I hope we may flatter ourselves we shall observe it together, you still young, and I not very old. You shall be the Urania to give a right direction to my telescope. What a vicissitude of things, replied the Marchioness, is there in this system! I am metamorphosed into a Urania, and supposed to be young at a time when it becomes unpolite to talk about years, and the non-appearance of a comet rendered more fatal than its appearance! It will appear too soon, answered I, to put us in rememberance of our past time, and our attraction. In this case, replied she, we may express ourselves contrary to the common saying,

'Tis expectation makes a blessing dear.

It is at present indeed a great happiness to be an astronomer. They at least expect nothing in vain; and how great a pleasure do they owe to this system, which gives them a full power over every thing in that heaven which is the object of their projects and desires!

Nothing, answered I, was a greater curiosity to astronomers, or more glorious for the Newtonian system, than the conjunction of Jupiter and Saturn, which happened in the beginning of the present age, an age so fertile in the most surprizing events. These two great planets were to approach each other, which the vast extent of their orbits, and the time employed in describing those orbits, had not very often suffered them to do.

If it could ever be hoped to see the effects of this mutual attraction in the disturbance and alterations in the motions of the planets, it was upon this occasion, when the two most powerful, in the whole solar system, approached each other, at a distance however of three hundred and fifty millions of miles. This was an observation in *great*, as decisive for the Newtonian celestial system as the experiments of refracting the coloured rays with a second prism, in order to prove whether colour was a modification of light or no, was in *little*. The curiosity in this affair was so much the greater, because the Newtonian system was then in its infancy; and time which gives strength to truth, and in which error vanishes away, had not yet decided any thing to the world in its favour.

The disturbance which Jupiter, the greatest of all the planets, occasioned in the motions of Saturn, and that which this planet reciprocally exercised upon the satellites of Jupiter, were so considerable that they could not escape the observations and testimony of astronomers, even those who were the least inclined to adopt the system, whom a difference of opinion from the wagers held against it, might easily induce to regard this phænomenon in a very superficial manner. And Sir Isaac Newton had the pleasure of extorting from his very enemies so strong and solemn a confirmation of his system. What are the triumphs of the Cæsars and Alexanders, those miserable conquerors who overturned two particles of this globe, when compared to the philosophical triumph of him who first discovered the vast extent of the universe?

Astronomy, said the Marchioness, has by this triumph amply rewarded Sir Isaac Newton for defending it so well in the affair of total eclipses. This mutual assistance, this commerce, if I may use the expression, of truth, must certainly be a very great honour to the sciences. This commerce, answered I, was never more evidently seen than in attraction. We may affirm, that every science, with a sort of emulation contributes to confirm this truth, just as the whole world anciently did to the raising the Roman empire.

Though I told you that the effects of attraction are more remarkable in the heavens than any where else, yet it is also very evident in all natural philosophy, hydrostatics, chemistry, and anatomy itself. Mr. Muscembrook, who even in philosophy presents the character of a true republican, confesses with that freedom that becomes a member of the Belgic state, that for the space of many years spent in the greatest variety of experiments, he has observed in all bodies certain motions and effects which could not be explained or underſtood by means of the external preſſure of any ambient fluid: but that nature proclaims aloud a law infuſed in bodies by which they are attracted, without a dependance upon impulſion. Chemical fermentations, the hardneſs of bodies, the round figure of drops of water, and of the earth itſelf, the ſeparation of the juices in the human body, the ſuction of water by ſpunges, its aſcent in thoſe tubes which from their extreme ſmallneſs are called *capillary*, and a thouſand other things, are inconteſtable arguments for this attraction. I believe that after ſo many repeated proofs you will permit me to introduce it triumphantly into optics, in order to explain the effects which depend on this mutual attraction of light and bodies. It would be very extraordinary, ſaid ſhe, if I ſhould refuſe to admit the mutual attraction of light and bodies, after I have ſeen the Sun and Saturn attract each other at ſo enormous a diſtance.

Not to ſay any thing more of diffraction, anſwered I, is not refraction an effect of this attractive power? Does it not ariſe from hence, that the mediums through which the light paſſes are indued with this force in a greater or leſs degree, according to the greater or leſs denſity of the medium? Otherwiſe the immenſe force of the earth which attracts every thing to herſelf, would render it impoſſible for any priſm, if it were as big as pike *Tenerif*, to attract the ſmalleſt ray of light.

While the light paſſes through the ſame medium, becauſe it is equally attracted on all ſides, it will not decline to any, but move forward according to that direction it received from the ſun or any other luminous body: if in its way it meets with another medium of a greater force, ſuch as glaſs for example compared to air, muſt it not decline towards this medium and immerse into it, approaching more or less to a perpendicular as the attraction of the new medium is more or less powerful?

In going out of glass into air, the light is again attracted by the air and the glass; but because the force of the glass is greater than that of the air, the light will remain behind the surface of the glass from whence it goes out, or behind that of the air into which it enters, and which immediately touches the glass itself.

Thus you see, how easily by the help of attraction is explained a phænomenon, which Des Cartes could not account for, unless by supposing that light could with greater facility pass through dense than rare mediums; which is in other words saying, that what makes the greatest resistance to all other bodies, must, by some other privilege of which I am ignorant, make the least resistance to this. It is surprising to see how all that experiments have discovered to happen in refractions, are geometrically deduced from this explication of the Newtonian philosophy.

To me, replied the Marchioness, who cannot enter into the sanctuary of the mathematics, it seems a sufficient proof that as the attractive force is greater in proportion as the density of the medium is so, the refraction must in that case be proportionably greater.

The Dutch, answered I, have found it to be much greater in Nova Zembla than here among us. The air is extremely cold, and consequently dense in this country, the habitation of white bears, and some Europeans, the miserable victims of the avarice or curiosity of their species.

By the help of this very great refraction they had the pleasure of seeing the sun after his long absence many days before the science of cosmography had permitted him to appear, and the density of the air, which generally oppresses and damps the spirits, served in this retreat of misery and darkness, to revive their imagination by an unexpectedly early light.

We may at present hope for more exact observations upon the density of the air and the refractions of this climate, which have never yet been examined by philosophical eyes. A learned company is now setting sail from France, to the Bothnic gulph, and another to Peru, in order by their united observations to determine if possible the true figure of the earth, and animated by the love of science, have the resolution to change the gardens and the delightful seats of pleasure in their own country, for the frozen rocks and desarts of Lapland.

In North America, the colds are incomparably more sharp than in Europe, at the same distance from the pole. There are in those seas mountains of ice of the same date perhaps as the world, among which are sometimes found ships at full sail as motionless as upon dry land.

Doctor Halley, whom the English nation regards with the highest respect as the friend and companion of Sir Isaac Newton, and whose thoughts are employed on no objects that are little or trifling, believes that these countries were once perhaps nearer the pole than they at present are; that a comet by giving a shock to the earth altered their situation, and by this means set them at a greater distance. But that notwithstanding this, the great magazine of ice formed before this terrible shock still remains, nor has the heat of following ages ever been able to melt it. Hence proceed the sharp colds and a stronger refraction caused by them.

On LIGHT and COLOURS. 261

Certain English sailors, who, above a century ago, endeavoured, without success, to find in North America a passage to the southern sea, were obliged to spend the winter in an island very little more north than London. Every thing there was transformed to ice, the house they had built, the sea, the ship, and even themselves.

They were obliged to cut the most spirituous wine with a hatchet, and the refraction was so strong, that they observed the rising moon of an oval figure extremely long, and the sun when at the horizon to be twice as big in breadth as in length. The air was sometimes so very clear in the depth of that severe winter, that they discovered more stars by two thirds than are usually seen, and the milky way appeared evidently to the naked eye, a collection of stars. Thus in these countries there would have been no need of a Democritus to conjecture it among the dreams of the ancient philosophy, nor a Galileo to verify it by the assistance of the telescope.

From a great number of experiments made in England, it evidently appears, that the refractive power of the air increases in proportion to its density, which is true likewise in other mediums which refract the light, but however with some exceptions. Air, water, and glass, sensibly observe this proportion. But oleaginous and sulphureous liquors, and which consequently are combustible, have a greater refraction than liquors of another nature even tho' they are more dense. Oil which is less dense than water, as appears by its swimming upon it, has however a greater force in refracting the light.

Alas! interrupted the Marchioness, I am a great enemy to exceptions, and I have a most mortal aversion to the *but* in conversation. Every one who takes it into his head to rail againſt our ſex before our very face, will doubtleſs except, with a conſtrained *but*, her who has the misfortune to be preſent. Satire, ſo agreeable to the malignity of our mind, becomes cold with theſe exceptions; our ſelf love is not ſufficiently flattered, and truth loſes too much when it becomes leſs general.

Exceptions of this ſort, anſwered I, are properly only new truths which ariſe from the diſcovery of many cauſes, which joined together generally concur to produce a certain effect. This greater refraction in a leſs denſity of medium ariſes from another particular correſpondence between theſe liquors and light. It acts upon them more than upon any other ſort, by agitating, warming and inflaming them more eaſily. It is juſt then, on the other hand, that theſe in return ſhould act more upon the light than other mediums do, by breaking and refracting it in a greater degree.

May we not conclude from hence that this force reſides chiefly in the ſulphureous parts of bodies? For this reaſon boiling water, in which theſe parts are more diſengaged, has a greater attractive force than cold water.

In general, warmth and rubbing augment the attractive force which is in bodies, or make it appear in a particular manner. Amber, all ſorts of pellucid gems, glaſs, hair, and many other things when they are rubbed, diſcover the force called *electrical*, and which is communicated to other bodies, carried to incredible diſtances, and whoſe effects are ſurprizing beyond all belief.

If a tub of glaſs be rubbed till it grows hot, it will attract light bodies, as leaves of gold or cotton, and afterwards drive them at a diſtance. It will raiſe a ſort of tempeſt in a heap of little pieces of burnt paper, by attracting and then tumultuously repelling them from itself. In short, this force is a species of magic wand, that communicates and awakens a power in bodies, which had before lain dormant and inactive.

A ball of ivory fastened to a cord of nine hundred or a thousand foot long, acquires the same power of attraction and repulsion, if the electrical tube be applied to the other end of the cord a thousand foot distant. You had very great reason, replied the Marchioness, to call this tube a sort of magic wand, for it really produces incomprehensible effects. At least, it is a mystery to me that it should with such rapidity draw the little bodies to itself, and afterwards with a sort of disdain remove and drive them away.

Observation, answered I, which has hitherto been our guide and clue in the intricate labyrinth of natural philosophy, will continue to give us the same assistance in that little way we have yet to go. It has conducted us to the discovery of new properties in light and colours, which have opened a new scene of optics to philosophy. It has conducted us to the discovery of attraction in the most secret retreats of bodies; which is likewise a new and surprizing quality of matter, by which all natural philpsophy is changed and renewed; and now this faithful guide leads us to *repulsion*, whose effects in nature are no less considerable and surprizing.

Are we not to impute it to this force, that flies are able to walk upon the water without wetting their legs, and that the particles, which fly off from bodies by means of heat or fermentation, are set at so great a distance from each other as to possess an infinitely greater space than they did at first?

The air after being compreſſed may be dilated to ſuch a degree as to poſſeſs a ſpace more than eight hundred twenty ſix thouſand times greater than it did when compreſſed, and this without being heated, which would dilate it ſtill more. That you may underſtand this force has no leſs influence in heaven than earth, the famous comet of 1682, approached ſo cloſe to the ſun that it was heated two thouſand times more than a red hot iron. The vapours ariſing from it, and caſt at a diſtance from each other by the repulſive force, adorned it with ſo formidable a tail that it took up in heaven the length of eighty million of Engliſh miles. It would have been very bad for us to have been near, and involved in it; for inſtead of gaining a ring or another moon, we ſhould have been calcined and burnt to aſhes, like a little ſtone in the focus of a burning glaſs.

Some perſons ſo taken up with the phantoms of the uncertain *future*, as not to ſee the fugitive *preſent*, expect that one day ſome comet will cauſe the univerſal conflagration of this globe. Comets have perhaps anciently produced a deluge, have ſtruck againſt the earth and overſet every thing in it, and who knows but one time or other they may bring a conflagration upon it, after which laying aſide its old ſpoils like the ſnake, it may again grow young and be renewed, and our great theatre change both it ſcenes and actors.

The preſent, replied ſhe, is ſo various and agreeable as it now ſtands, that I am greatly deceived, if it may not divert us as yet a long time without any change.

But perhaps it is to theſe comets that we are obliged for one of the fineſt changes, and what we every day enjoy. They are perhaps the ingenious mechanicks that have rendered our theatre capable of being turned round like that of Curio, so famous in antiquity, where the Roman people, the conquerors of the world, the race of heroes, and the portion granted to mankind by the immortal gods, sat upon a frail machine, in which they could not even applaud their public shews without danger. We at present perhaps owe to some comet, without apprehending any calamitous accident, the rotation of our earth, the perpetual and constant succession of light and shadow; in short, the pleasing variety of day and night. One of these perhaps by giving us a shock has occasioned this motion in us as well as the other planets which are discovered to be endowed with it.

Before this we had, like the cold inhabitants of the pole, six months day and six months night, but without gaining like them either a strong refraction or a long twilight to anticipate and prolong our day. A little moon-light would from time to time have faintly illuminated that long and melancholy darkness. What optics, what colours could we ever have had for six continued months, unless the comet with its shock had lent us its assistance? Since every thing, replied the Marchioness, stands well at present, heaven guard us for the future from the proximity of any one of them, from the shocks, the conflagrations and the deluge with which they menace us, and from that repulsive force that renders them so very formidable. But are not these the riddles as well as terrors of natural philosophy, that the same bodies should be both attracted and repelled?

I do not know, answered I, after some pause, whether I ought to introduce you any farther into the sanctuary of the Newtonian philosophy. There are in this certain my-

DIALOGUE VI.

steries still deeper and more sublime than those to which you have already been admitted. You should now invoke those spirits the first-born sons of light, the guardians of those secret truths which they imparted to our philosopher, that they would suffer me to discover to you things concealed from the sight of mortals, and deeply immersed in a gloomy mist and the most profound night. You must now entirely divest yourself of those few remains of profaneness which may still attend you. Tell me, Madam, what courage do you feel for truth? The same, answered she, that a brave soldier feels to follow his captain wherever valour calls. I follow you without fear wherever truth leads the way.

You appear, answered I, to think it a riddle in philosophy, that the same bodies should be both attracted and repelled; and indeed there is some reason for your thinking so. But would not the riddle be still greater, if I tell you that these two contrary forces, the attractive and repulsive, are of the same nature, and in short it is only the same force which discovers itself in different manners and various circumstances? The Marchioness, at this, could scarce forbear laughing. What! said she, do you call the attractive and repulsive force the same thing? One acts directly contrary to the other, since the first attracts and the last repels. Are these those sublime mysteries in natural philosophy, of which you hardly thought me worthy, and which you have introduced with so much apparatus? Does not all this greatly resemble the physician in Moliere, who affirmed roast and boiled to be the same thing.

What! answered I, do you ridicule the most sacred things in natural philosophy, and of whose use you are yet ignorant? What a spirit of profaneness still remains in you! but you shall quickly be punished. Remember the conclusion which you yourself just now deduced from that very attraction you made so great a difficulty to admit. Ladies of all persons have least reason to be surprized that the same thing should produce contrary effects. Do not the highest reserve and an evident partiality often proceed from the same principle, and teach connoisseurs to draw the same conclusion from them? The sun hardens and softens according to the different circumstances in which he exercises his heat.

This truth is no less evident in the most noisy affairs of human life, than in the phænomena of gallantry and natural philosophy. The same thirst of leaving an empty name and living in the imaginary breath of posterity, burnt the temple at Ephesus in Asia, and precipitated a Roman and his horse into an open gulph in the midst of the forum at Rome. The same passion made Curtius an hero, and Erostratus an incendiary.

There are certain things which to the vulgar, nay even the philosophical vulgar, may appear as evident contradictions in the same man, whom some upon that account have imagined to be double, as others did the governor of the universe, so that what the one willed, the other disapproved: but are not these contradictions the necessary consequences of the same passion and the same motives?

Thus the very same cause, by which bodies are attracted, may in some circumstances repel them. There are found certain analogies between these two forces, which give us great reason to conclude that they are in reality only the same force which produces different effects.

It is generally found that where the attractive force is

weak, the repulsive too is weak, and where the one is strong the other is strong also. Refraction which depends on one of these two forces, and reflection on the other, are both effected where there is a surface that separates two bodies of different density. For while the rays proceed in the same medium, and do not meet with one of a different density, they are neither reflected nor refracted.

Those rays, which are most refrangible, are likewise more easily reflected than the rest. In bodies by which the light is more refracted, it is likewise more strongly reflected. And in general where the attracted force is greatest, the reflective and repulsive is greatest also. Diamonds, which refract the light very strongly, give it in proportion a stronger reflection. Hence proceed the vivacity of their colours and their fine sparkling lustre.

These analogies, replied the Marchioness, are very pretty and very good, and so are the examples by which you introduced them, and very strongly reproach my rashness. I am heartily penitent for my fault in laughing, when I should have admired, and despising what I ought to have regarded with veneration. But did not you tell me that reflection happens when light meets with the solid parts of bodies, and is from thence repelled? This explication seemed very intelligible to me, and perhaps more so than what you at present intimate.

It is Des Cartes, Madam, who gave you this explication, and not I, therefor you may be in some apprehensions about it. An ingenious author gives a very useful piece of advice, that in philosophy we should be as diffident of what we imagine ourselves to understand very easily, as of what we do not understand at all.

If refraction was made when the light meets with the

solid parts of bodies, as you so clearly understand it ought to be, do you know what an inconvenience would from thence arise in nature? you would no longer have either toilette or looking-glasses.

A surface, however smooth and polished it may be, is however full of protuberances and sensible irregularities discoverable by a microscope. Imagine all bodies which you believe the most smooth and polished, to be like water when it is rufled by the wind. The light must be reflected from all bodies irregularly as it is from water thus rufled, and could never be sent back with that regularity as is necessary for you to see yourself in a looking glass. Is not this paying a great price for your fine explication? Is it really true, answered she, that it will cost so dear? Perhaps you put me into a greater terror than the danger deserves. Is it not possible that these irregularities in the surfaces of glasses, though sensible to the microscope, may yet be insensible to the light?

You are grown extremely difficult, Madam, answered I. The protuberances and cavities in the most smooth and polished glasses, are when compared to a particle of light, what the Alps or Pyrenees would be in respect of a tennis-ball. The irregularities of a looking-glass are discoverable by common microscopes, but there is no microscope so perfect as to shew the pores of diamond, through which the light however passes very copiously. It would be a terrible circumstance for us, if the particles of light were not almost infinitely small. The force of bodies is reckoned from the quantity of matter that they contain, which is called the mass, and from their velocity; the greater therefor their mass and velocity, the greater is their force.

DIALOGUE VI.

The particles of light have an incredible velocity, for they come from the sun to the earth in about eight minutes, and thus in eight minutes they run through a space of eighty one million of miles. Their velocity then being so extremely great as to exceed more than ten million times that of the swiftest English horses, their mass must be almost infinitely small, or else a single particle of light, instead of animating and reviving all nature by its appearance, would produce upon our earth the most terrible effects of a cannon.

The good effects, answered the Marchioness, of that diffidence we ought to shew to men, extend likewise to philosophers; for by this means the one gives greater proofs of what we desire should be true, and the other of what really is so. I will for the future be very careful not to believe you too hastily.

For this time at least, answered I, you cannot accuse yourself of too much credulity. It will never burthen your conscience that you have not had sufficient arguments to believe that reflection is not made by the meeting of light with the solid parts of bodies. For besides the great inconvenience which would arise if this supposition were true, observation informs us, that light, transmitted through a piece of glass, suffers a stronger reflection at going out of the glass than it did at entering into it. Now how is it possible that light should find more solid parts in the air than in the glass itself, to occasion this stronger reflection?

Besides, if water or oil be placed immediately behind the glass, the reflection becomes weaker. Will the light find fewer solid parts in water or oil than in air?

Lastly, if the air which is behind the glass be taken away by an instrument made for that purpose, the reflection will be much stronger than it was before the air was removed. Will you say that light meets with a greater number of solid parts in a vacuum than in the air? Heaven forbid that I should say it, replied the Marchioness; I will rather make the repulsive force to be the cause of reflection. In these cases, answered I, it is not the repulsive but the attractive force. When a ray goes out of the glass into air, it is attracted by the air and the glass; hence that part of it, which was nearest the glass, returns back as if it had been reflected; if the air be entirely taken away, this part being extremely attracted by the glass, and hardly any thing by what remains after the air is removed, it returns back again almost entire.

But if water or oil, which attract the ray much more strongly than the air does, be placed behind the glass, a less part of the ray will return back than there did while the air remained. Lastly, when the forces of the two mediums are balanced, as for instance, if a liquor be applied to the glass of pretty near the same density, or another piece of glass, the ray must pass entire, and there will be no reflection.

In general, we may affirm that the attractive force is the cause of the reflection of the rays, when the light passes from a dense into a rare medium; and the repulsive, when it passes from a rare to a dense.

In both cases, since the attractive and repulsive force are propagated at some distance from bodies, the light is reflected notwithstanding its distance from the reflecting body. Just as when it begins to be refracted, it is somewhat distant from the refracting medium, in the same manner as it is from the extremity of bodies when passing near them, it is turned out of its direct path and curved by diffraction. Hence you see that solid parts and Des Cartes's explication have less to do with reflection than ever.

Poor Des Cartes, continued she, is attacked in his very last retrenchments. There is nothing wanting to complete his overthrow but for us to assert, that as light is not reflected from solid parts, so neither is it transmitted from the pores of bodies; and thus he may return back like that momentaneous Alexander of the north, who, after the most rapid and noisy victories, at length lost the best of his own dominions.

In order to deny him every thing, and give him leave to return home as soon as he pleases, we will at least deny that the quantity or magnitude of the pores in bodies, contributes any thing to their transparency. It is proved on the contrary, that if the pores of a body, for instance, paper, be filled with water or oil, it loses its opacity, and becomes transparent; whereas if the pores in a body be multiplied, as when glass is reduced to powder, it loses its transparency and becomes opaque.

It is in homogeneity we are to seek the cause of transparency. If there be many pores in a body, and these be filled with a matter different from that of the body itself, the light will meet with a thousand reflections and refractions in the internal parts, and thus it will be utterly extinguished. The air ceases to be transparent when it is cloudy, though it is then lighter than when it is clear, and consequently more porous. Its opacity can rise from no other cause but that it is at that time heterogenous, which makes the rays that pass through it suffer innumerable reflections and refractions, by which means they are very soon stifled and extinguished. Thus the froth of Champagne is opaque, though much more porous and lighter than the wine itself.

This seems to furnish us with an argument to infer, that the heavens cannot be filled with matter however rare it be supposed, even if all contained within the vast orb of Saturn, and though its pores should be as small as you can possibly conceive, it might, after being perfectly united so as to leave no empty space, be grasped in one hand.

What strange relation is this you tell me? replied the Marchioness. Is the Newtonian philosophy some golden fleece which we must not undertake the conquest of, till we have first passed through a thousand strange portents, and subdued a thousand monsters of imagination.

Do you believe, answered I, that gold the precious substance for which mankind do and suffer so much, and for which we feel the greatest thirst when we ought to be most satisfied, gold I say, and diamonds themselves, the most shining work of nature, notwithstanding their great weight and gravity, contain a great quantity of matter? It will appear strange when I tell you how very little that quantity really is when compared to that vacuum between the parts, and which to our deluded eye seems perfectly full.

The solid parts, contained in a piece of glass, are no more considered with regard to its extent, than a grain of sand to the terraqueous globe. It is very surprizing how little solid matter there is in the world, and with how few materials, if I may use that expression, it is built. Perhaps if you knew the truth you would be afraid you walked upon cotton, and were in danger of crushing it under your feet, even if they were as light as those of the swift Camilla.

Now if the matter of the heavens be imagined unconceivably rare and subtle, yet the light, which, notwithstanding its prodigious velocity, employs according to the last calculations six years in coming from the stars to us, must be intirely extinguished by that multiplicity of reflections and refractions which it must suffer in that immense passage; just as a numerous and flourishing army, in a long march, must decrease and perish by the fatigues and obstacles it meets upon the road.

I see with pleasure, said the Marchioness, how the properties of our light conduct us to empty heaven, and after having set the earth in motion, to clear its way. The diffractions too, answered I, which the light would suffer from the particles of this celestial matter, would contribute not a little to extinguish it, in the same manner as they would do in bodies that are very porous and heterogeneous. It is surprizing that in the notes which Perrault wrote upon Vitruvius, he seems, if I remember right, to have had some faint notion of this truth. Rarefraction, said he, that is, a distance of parts, renders bodies opaque, because these which were at first homogeneal, when rarefied, become heterogeneous.

It seems much more surprizing, said the Marchioness, that any person could clearly see and demonstrate that two things so very opposite as reflection and refraction should yet arise from the same cause: this I must confess will always be a wonder to me.

The facility, answered I, and the obstacles which the light meets in passing out of one medium into another, are almost in the same case. Perhaps an exceedingly subtile fluid diffused in the confines of the mediums, extremely quick in its vibrations, and in which the light by percussion excites an undulating and tremulous motion, as a stone does in water, or a voice in the air, is the cause of both the facility and obstacles in question. Thus if the light happens to be in the concavity of the waves of this fluid, it passes freely through it, but if in their summit, it is drove back again.

Hence come the *fits of easy transmission and refraction*, that is, the same ray of light is in one moment transmitted, and in the next reflected; and because the vibrations of this fluid are exceedingly rapid, the rays appear to us both transmitted and reflected at the same time.

But we are now arrived to the confines of nature, where our ideas grow dark and confused: these are the barriers of knowlege, beyond which no force of human faculties is permitted to proceed. I myself perhaps have run too great a length.

Sir Isaac Newton, under the form of questions, proposed many things which are probably the recesses where nature withdraws to conceal herself from mortal eyes. The analogy betwixt sound and colour, the strange metamorphoses of light into bodies, and bodies into light, the two-fold and surprizing refractions of island chrystal, rock chrystal, and that sort lately discovered in Brasil, will always be impenetrable enigmas to mankind, since this Oedipus was not able to solve them.

How very different from the modest doubts of this legislator of the wise are the rash assertions of the seducers of the multitude. These however promise those very men, whom they have always deceived with the same flatteries, to open the temple of truth so often tried in vain, in the most expeditious and easy manner by the help of certain new principles; just as others with certain new systems of their own spread artful nets for human avarice, and promife at once to enrich a nation which they have always impoverifhed by the very fame fchemes. The pleafing and vain delufion of hope leads fome in hafte to the *bank*, others to the academy. The beginning of an affair is generally agreeable to our flattering expectations. The wind is commonly favourable to the fhip juft loofed from the port, and two bright eyes give an agreeable invitation at the firft appearance. The bank by converting hopes at firft into gold preferves and increafes its reputation; and philofophy by judicious prefaces maintains its honours, more fuccefsful in banifhing old errors, than fubftituting new truths in their place. Thus they, who by a prudent diffidence foon extricated themfelves from the fnare, either brought back a reputable increafe of their fortune, or were rationally delivered from their paft prejudices. But there are very few fo wife as not to lofe the prefent in forming projects for the future, or not to make the happinefs of to-day, a ftep to the mifery of to-morrow. The cheat at length is difcovered, and the firft are left with their fcrutoirs, full of notes worth nothing, while the laft have their heads embarraffed with notions of preffure, rotations, globules and vortices, the falfe coin of philofophy. Sir Ifaac Newton, guided by a flow yet fure experience, promifes no more than what experience is able to perform. Where that leaves him he ftops; by its affiftance he diftinguifhes truth from falfhood, evidence from probability, and in the extent of his *own*, difcovers the limits of the *human* underftanding.

Are not the rays of light, fays Sir Ifaac Newton, very fmall bodies of different fizes, the leaft of which make violet, the weakeft and darkeft of all the colours, and more eafily diverted by the attractive force of the *prifm* from the right path? And the reft, as they are bigger and bigger, make the ftronger and more lucid colours, blue, green, yellow and red, and are more difficultly refracted, in proportion to the greater ftrength of the colours, and the larger fize of the bodies that compofe them?

It is certain that the rays of light differ from each other in colour, refrangibility, and the force with which they ftrike our fenfes. Scarlet dazzles the fight, the azure of heaven languidly moves it, and the verdure of a meadow ftrikes it with a very pleafing fenfation.

Only one of thefe differences, faid the Marchionefs, had been fufficient to make an ordinary philofopher put an abfolute difference in the fize of the particles of light, whereas two or three are hardly enough to fupply ours with a conjecture.

In the vaft and unlimited perfpective of nature, anfwered I, there are objects that we are for ever condemned to fee languid and confufed, without hoping that any telefcope can make them appear either lefs diftant or more diftinct. The moderation of our philofopher, in never affirming any thing to be true which was not demonftrated by obfervation, may ferve for an example to the moft rafh afferters. Who could have more reafon to think himfelf capable of afcending heaven, or bringing the fecrets of nature in triumph from thence, than Sir Ifaac Newton, who, poifed upon the wings of geometry, could take his flight through immenfe fpaces, till then impenetrable to human curiofity?

What a ftrange condition, replied the Marchionefs, is ours! We know what fize in a particle at a great diftance from our fight is neceffary to reflect a certain colour; but, what is this colour itfelf which we have always immediately before our eyes? Hardly can we form any idea of it by a feeble conjecture: In one cafe we have the fight of a lynx, in the other we are abfolutely blind. There our fenfes are refined beyond what we could have expected; here they feem to abandon us all at once.

There are fome perfons, anfwered I, who have believed that the many difficulties which attend our little degree of knowlege, the great number of fyftems, the various emblems of human ignorance, and that continual tantalizing which philofophers fuffer in their fearching after truth, proceed from no other caufe than our want of a fixth natural fenfe which might reveal a great part of what is at prefent hid from us, and efcapes perhaps thofe five fenfes given us by nature to lay hold on external objects, and bring them to the mind.

As there are certain animals among us, who, by virtue of fenfes, of which we perhaps have no knowlege, forefee the change of the feafons, and approach of the morning, and, without having read Diofcorides or any other botanift, can amidft a thoufand others diftinguifh that falutary herb that cures their hurts; who knows but in fome other fyftem, in the world of Jupiter perhaps, there may be animals which, more fharp fighted than our philofophers, may difcover the fize of thofe particles that compofe the variety of colours, and in what manner, without the affiftance of ropes or pullies, they may attract Saturn at a diftance of more than three hundred and fifty millions of miles?

But in return, as in that planet, which is not depopulated by the race of war, the inhabitants have no idea of the pleafures of love, fo, according to the agreeable hiftorian of thefe worlds, every thing is diverfified, and put in a juft balance; thofe people, who are thoroughly acquainted with the nature of colours, may perhaps want the fenfe proper to give them a perception of the moft agreeable harmony of thofe colours upon the cheeks of their *Chloes*; and though, perfectly fkilled in the attractions of the planets, are perhaps infenfible to the more pleafing attractions of beauty, which are preferable to any fpeculation whatever.

But however it be with regard to our prefent fpeculation, the moft vain perhaps of all others, it is not for our advantage to feek occafions to put us in mind of our defects, nor be fo ingenious in tormenting ourfelves. We fhall not be deftitute of either knowlege or pleafure, if we make a good ufe of the fenfes fallen to our lot. Though you know nothing wherein confifts the nature of light and colours but by conjecture, there will not perhaps be wanting fome perfons to affirm you know much more of it than is proper for a lady. The fault will be thrown entirely upon me, who upon thofe few verfes which give occafion to our fubject, have made you a comment long enough for a poem upon the Newtonian philofophy. It will be well for it, if you diffemble your knowlege with thofe perfons who ridicule what they ought to learn, and if to the fcience of natural philofophy you join that of the world.

What, cried the Marchionefs, am I fo learned that I ought to ftudy to be ignorant? May I venture ferioufly to call myfelf a Newtonian? You have already renounced your philofophical errors, anfwered I. The light of Newtonianifm has diffipated the Cartefian phantoms which deluded your fight. You are now really a Newtonian, and it is no fmall advantage to *truth* that you are fo. I will fome time give a hiftory of the fine conqueft I have acquired for her, and I am certain if I could give a juſt deſcription of my fair diſciple, my book would never want readers nor true philoſophy a numerous train of proſelytes. You ſhall be the Venus that muſt lend the agreeable Ceſtus to this auſtere Juno, and give her thoſe attractive charms that will render her engaging and amiable to mankind.

THE END.

Miſtakes to be rectified.

Page 73. line 18. *for* : not, *read* . Not.
ib. l. 31. *for* . Did, *read* ; did.
81. l. 7. *for* deeper, *read* higher.
180. l. 10. *for* article, *read* Ancile.
205. l. 8. *for* not, *read* and.
227. l. 2. *for* barel, *read* barely.
257. l. 11. *for* particles, *read* parts.
ib. l. 28. *for* preſents, *read* preſerves.
261. l. 27. *for* even though they are more denſe, *read* even though they are more denſe than the oils.

BOOKS printed and sold by ROBERT URIE, at his Printing Office, foot of the Saltmarket.

I. An Essay on Painting. Translated from the Italian of Count Algarotti. This elegant performance consists of the following articles, viz. Introduction. Of the first education of a painter. Of perspective. Of symmetry. Of colouring. Of the camera obscura. Of drapery. Of landscape and architecture. Of the costume. Of Invention. Of disposition. Of the expression of the passions. Of proper books for a painter. Of a friend. Of the importance of the public judgment. Of the criticism necessary to a painter. Of the painter's balance. Of Imitation. Of the recreations of a painter. Of the fortunate condition of a painter. Conclusion. 12mo. price 2 s. 6 d. bound.

II. Miscellaneous pieces in literature, history, and philosophy. By Mr. d' Alembert, member of the royal accademy of Inscriptions at Paris. This elegant book contains the following articles. Remarks on Translation. A discourse before the French Academy. Reflections on elocution, and style in general. The abuse of Criticism in religion. An Essay upon the alliance betwixt learned men and the great. Reflections on the use and abuse of philosophy in matters that are properly relative to taste. A short account of the government of Geneva. Memoirs of Christina, queen of Sweden. 12mo. price 3 s. bound.

III. Cosmotheoros: Or, conjectures concerning the planets and their inhabitants. Translated from the Latin of the celebrated Christian Huygens. A new edition corrected, and illustrated with plates. 12mo. price 2 s. bound.

IV. The poetical works of John Dyer, L L. B. Containing 1. The Fleece, a poem in four books. 2. A poem on Grongar hill. 3. The Ruins of Rome, a poem. 12mo. price 2 s. bound.

V. The philosophical works of William Dudgeon, Esq; Consisting of the following pieces. 1. The state of the moral world considered; or a vindication of providence in the government of the moral world. 2. A letter to the Author of the state of the moral world considered. Wherein some satisfying account is attempted to be given of the nature of virtue and vice, the origin of moral evil, and the end and duration of future punishment. 3. A Catechism: collected by a father for the use of his children. 4. A view of the Necessitarian or best scheme, freed from the objections of Mr. Crousaz, in his examination of Pope's essay on man. 5. Philosophical letters concerning the being and attributes of God. 12mo. price 3 s. bound.

VI. A treatise on religious toleration. Occasioned by the execution of the unfortunate John Calas: unjustly condemned and broken upon the wheel at Thoulouse, for the supposed murder of his own son. By Mr. de Voltaire, 2mo. price 2 s. 6 d bound.

VII. The Newtonian philosophy compared with that of Leibnitz. In which not only the sentiments and opinions of those two eminent philosophers, but also of Des Cartes, Locke, Dr. Clark, Collins, and Spinosa, concerning the existence of a Deity, space, duration, liberty, goodness of the divine administration, immateriality of the soul, matter, etc. are all impartially compared and examined. 12mo. price 1 s. in boards

VIII. Dialogues, and essays, literary and philosophical, etc. 12mo. price 2 s. 6 d. bound.

IX. An Essay on an active and contemplative life; and when and why the one ought to be preferred to the other. 12mo. price 1 s. in boards.

X. Dialogues concerning Education. Betweena Courtier, a Lawyer, a Soldier, a country Gentleman, an Alderman, and a Bishop. 12mo. Price 1 s. in boards.

XI. The history of the conquests and discoveries of the English in North America and the West Indies. Containing an accurate account of all our settlements, their soil, produce, and commerce, both in America, and in the West Indies. 12mo. Price bound 2 s. 6 d.

XII. The history of the life of the celebrated Agricola, the first Roman general that conquered Scotland. With an account of the situation, climate, and people of Britain, at that time. Translated from the Latin of Tacitus, by Thomas Gordon, Esq; author of Cato's letters, Independent Whig, etc. 12mo. price stitched 1 s.

XIII. Sermons on the following important subjects, viz. On the Trinity. On mutual subjection. On the testimony of conscience. On brotherly love. The difficulty of knowing one's self. On false witness. On the poor man's contentment. On the causes of the wretched condition of Ireland. Upon sleeping in church. By the Reverend Dr. Swift, Dean of St. Patrick's Dublin. 12mo. price bound 3 s.

XIV. Devotions, and forms of prayer. I. for particular persons. II. for a family. By the reverend Dr. Benjamin Hoadly, late lord bishop of Winchester. 12mo. price 1 s. stitched.

XV. The complete songster: or, a new tea table miscellany. Being the most choice collection of Scotch and English songs in the British language. 12mo. Price 2 s. bound.

XVI. The history of the republic of Florence, in eight books. Translated from the Italian of the celebrated Machiavel, secretary to the republic.——N. B. This history comprehends the whole transactions of Florence, intermixed with the affairs of the other Italian states, from its rise, down to the death of Lorenzo the Great, the father of learning, and the patron of arts and sciences, that under his and his son's protection, the famous pope, Leo X. flourished in such perfection, at that time, in Italy, and were from thence communicated, in some degree, to the other kingdoms of Europe. 2 vol. 12mo. Price 5 s. bound.

XVII. The life of Gustavus Adolphus, king of Sweden. From the French of the celebrated Monf. Bayle, author of the historical and critical dictionary. 12mo. Price 2 s. 6 d. bound.

XVIII. The history of the revolutions in Portugal. 12mo. Price 2 s. bound.

XIX. The history of the revolution in Sweden, occasioned by the changes of religion, and alteration of the government in that kingdom. 12mo. Price 3 s. bound.

The above two translated from the French of the celebrated Abbe de Vertot.

www.ingramcontent.com/pod-product-compliance
Lightning Source LLC
Chambersburg PA
CBHW032121230426
43672CB00009B/1816